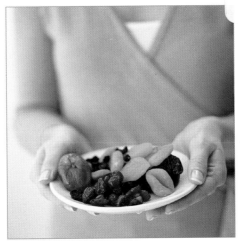

EAT ALL DAY **DIET**

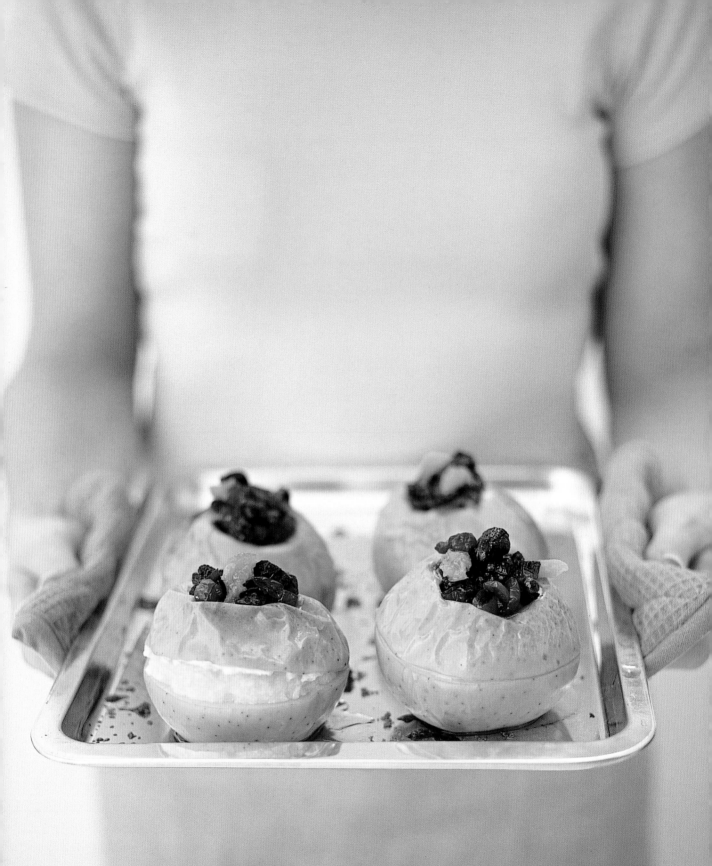

hamlyn

EAT ALL DAY DIET

Eat 6 meals a day and lose weight fast!

HELEN FOSTER

First published in Great Britain in 2007 by Hamlyn,
a division of Octopus Publishing Group Ltd,
2–4 Heron Quays, London E14 4JP

Copyright © Octopus Publishing Group Ltd 2007

Distributed in the United States and Canada by
Sterling Publishing Co., Inc.
387 Park Avenue South, New York, NY 10016-8810

ISBN-13: 978-0-600-59284-6
ISBN: 0-600-59284-7

A CIP catalogue record for this book is available
from the British Library

Printed and bound in China

10 9 8 7 6 5 4 3 2 1

This book is meant to be used as a general
reference and recipe guide to aid weight loss.
However, you are urged to consult a health-care
professional to check whether it is a suitable
weight loss plan for you, before embarking on it.

While all reasonable care has been taken during the
preparation of this edition, neither the publishers,
editors, nor the author can accept responsibility
for any consequences arising from the use of
this information.

NOTES
This books includes dishes made with nuts and
nut derivatives. It is advisable for those with
known allergic reactions to nuts and nut
derivatives and those who may be potentially
vulnerable to these allergies, such as pregnant and
nursing mothers, invalids, the elderly, babies and
children, to avoid dishes made with nuts and nut
oils. It is also prudent to check the labels of
preprepared ingredients for the possible inclusion
of nut derivatives.

Meat and poultry should be cooked thoroughly. To
test if poultry is cooked, pierce the flesh through
the thickest part with a skewer or fork — the juices
should run clear, never pink or red. All the recipes
in this book have been analyzed by a professional
nutritionist. The analysis refers to each serving.

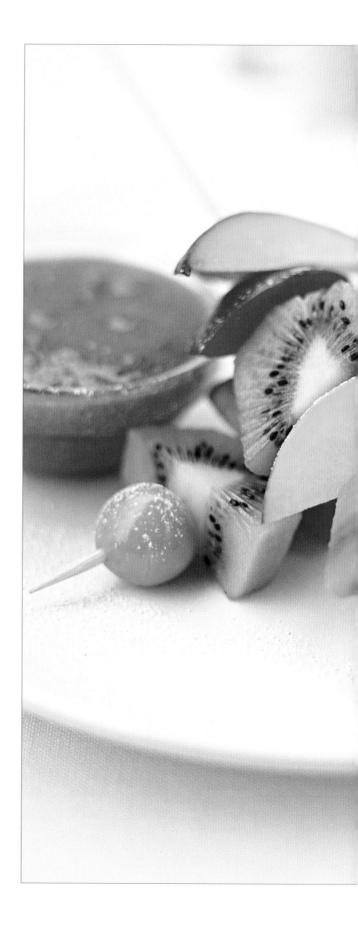

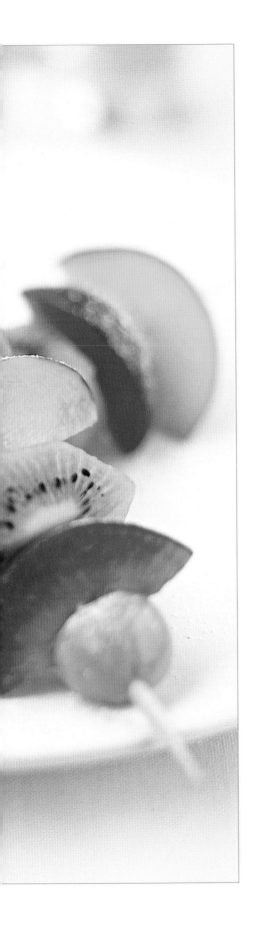

Contents

1
2
3
4
5
6

Introduction

Whether you are thumbing through this book in a bookstore or library, or you have already bought a copy and are at home taking your first steps to your new weight-loss regime, there is probably one big question going through your mind: "How is it possible to eat all day long and lose weight?"

For most of us, eating three square meals a day has become a thing of the past. Unlike past generations, who sat down and ate their breakfast, lunch, and dinner every day, most of us rush our meals if we eat them at all. We focus primarily on quickly digested foods high in refined carbohydrates that we can eat while we multitask. When our energy plummets a few hours later, we then rev things up with regular doses of sugary or chocolate treats and some caffeine. The result is that lifestyle experts now refer to us as the grazing generation, and the average person now eats five or six times a day.

However, snacking tends to stop when we want to lose weight. We either try an eating plan that involves eating only, say, protein or cabbage soup, or we decide to eat sensibly by cutting out all those in-between meal snacks. And, then, three days into the plan we find ourselves quitting in misery after spending another day fixating on the clock as we try to ignore the rumbling of our stomachs. The truth is, given our current busy lives, switching to a regime without snacks just doesn't make good lifestyle sense.

It is clear why we do snack, however. Many of the foods we choose to snack on come packed with fat, salt, and sugar. The result is that snacking is now the primary source of excess calories in our diets and therefore most often linked to weight gain. However, done in the right way, snacking can be an incredibly powerful weight-loss tool. Eating between meals can actually make you slim if you do it correctly — and that is what this book is all about.

You will find out how, by snacking in the right way three times a day and combining this with three small meals, you can create a stream of biological changes in your system that makes weight loss easier than ever before. You will be able to do it without hunger pangs, energy slumps, or that constant fixation with forbidden foods that you experience on traditional diet plans, and you could also transform your health from within.

The diet explained

The principle of this weight-loss plan is that you are going to be eating three low-calorie meals and three nutrient-filled snacks at two- to three-hour intervals throughout the day. Instead of skipping meals to lose weight or eating the traditional three square meals with no snacks in between you are going to be eating six times a day and still lose weight.

The reason this can happen is because eating six times a day influences the speed at which you burn calories each day; in other words, it alters your metabolic rate. It does this in two ways: regular eating prevents the slowdown in metabolism that usually occurs when you cut calories; it also maximizes the amount of energy you burn each day via a process called *thermogenesis* which revs up your metabolism every time you eat. This, combined with a healthy eating plan that controls the amount of calories/kilojoules you consume, maximizes the deficit in energy you need to burn fat and lose weight.

Eating this way also helps you lose weight as it prevents the hunger pangs that can destroy traditional diets but it also fundamentally alters the balance of various weight-loss/fat-storing hormones in the body. While you are on this particular plan, your body exists in a state more conducive to weight loss than it would be on a more traditional type of diet.

Exactly how all this happens is explained fully on the following ten pages but for now remember this one thing — 1500 calories eaten over five or six meals and snacks a day are more diet-friendly than those same 1500 calories consumed over two or three meals. This simple fact could explain why researchers at the University of Massachusetts found that people who eat at least four times are day are 45 percent less likely to be overweight than those who eat three or less meals a day, and why researchers at the University of Michigan discovered that the more frequently people ate, the lower their weight and body measurements were likely to be. Simply eating more often can help you get in shape and stay that way for life.

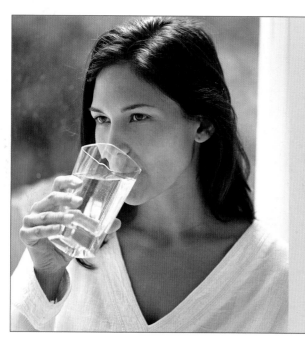

Craving countdown

If you get an uncontrollable craving for something else before or even after you snack don't give in. Just try to distract yourself for ten minutes — that's how long the average food craving lasts and if you can get past this point without eating you'll have successfully avoided temptation for another day. Even better, spend that ten minutes sipping a glass of water or herbal tea — remember, many of us mistake food cravings for thirst.

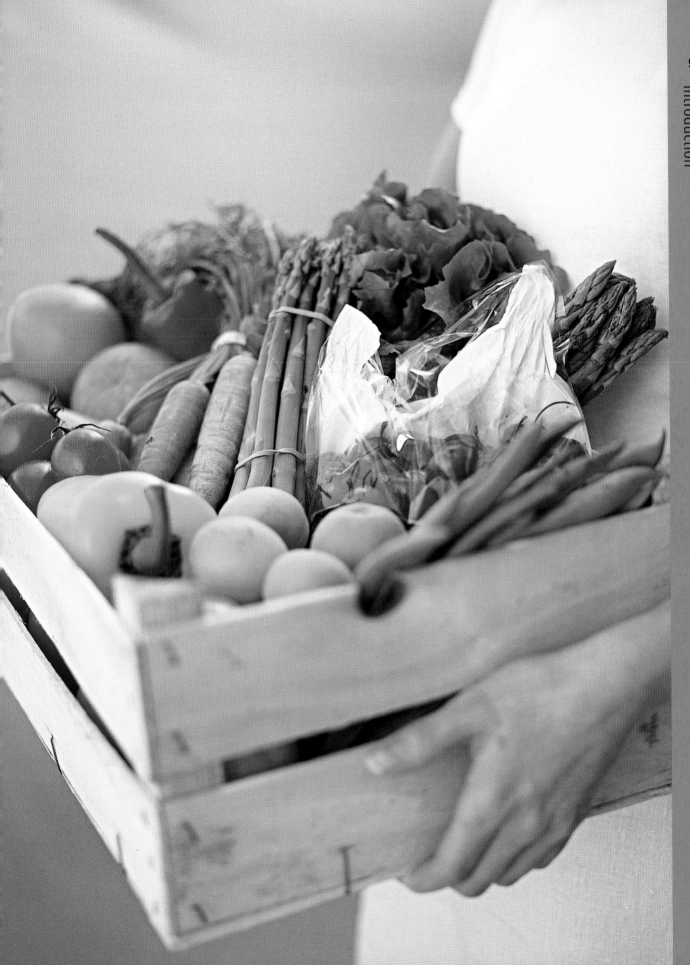

How frequent eating affects metabolism

While most of us believe that eating is something that only puts calories into the body, in fact, ten percent of the calories we burn up each day are used when we eat — chewing, digesting, and the assimilation of nutrients from our food is actually a pretty labor intensive process. As a result, our metabolic rate increases every single time we consume a meal or snack, and by switching it on more often throughout the day (as you do by eating little and often) you maximize the amount of calories that you can burn every 24 hours.

Exactly how fast your metabolic rate increases after eating depends on the types of food you eat. Protein, for example, will speed things up by up to 30 percent, fiber boosts the rate by around 15 percent while a meal containing solely fat will only raise the metabolic rate by two or three percent. Thankfully, not many of us will snack on a stick of butter or teaspoon of oil only, which means that on this frequent-eating plan, every meal you eat will trigger a moderate to high metabolic burst that can last up to two hours after you've eaten. The result is that your body is constantly running at an increased metabolic rate, and you are continually burning the calories you need to lose weight. But increasing calorie burn isn't the only way that frequent consumption can increase metabolism speed.

More muscle means less fat

On many diets, particularly those promising weight loss of more than $2^1/_4$ lb a week, not only does your metabolism slow down because you cut calories (see box opposite), but the weight you lose does not come solely from your fat stores but from the loss of lean muscle tissue. Muscle is what fitness experts call metabolically active, meaning that it burns calories even when you are sitting still, so by losing muscle you actively slow down your metabolism.

When you eat frequently, this muscle-stripping effect doesn't occur. Researchers at Japan's Nagoya University put two sets of dieters on the same diet of 1200 calories (5040 kj), but asked one set to consume them in two large meals, and another set to have six mini meals. The researcher concluded that the frequent eaters lost more body fat and retained more muscle than those who were eating the larger meals. Numerous other studies have also confirmed these results, proving conclusively that eating little and often preserves muscle mass. This means that not only do you lose weight more easily; it also makes it more likely that you'll keep that weight off when you reach your desired goal.

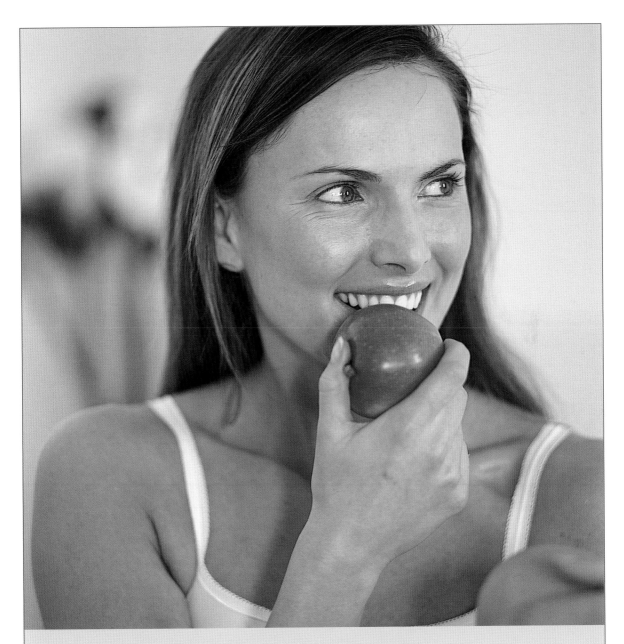

What happens to your metabolism when you cut calories

Although we live in the 21st century, our physiology is still that of our caveman ancestors. When you decide to go on a low-calorie diet, your body thinks that famine is coming and that it had better conserve as much energy in the form of high-calorie body fat as it can. As a result, your metabolism starts to slow and you burn fewer calories. So if a woman weighing 185 lb goes on a 1000-calorie (4200 kj) a day diet, her metabolism will slow by roughly 400 calories

(1680 kj) a day, and only 800 (3360 kj) of those calories will actually contribute to weight loss.

By eating little and often you trick your body out of this process. Even though you are cutting calories and losing weight, the body doesn't feel as if food is scarce because it is getting regular injections of energy and nutrients. This prevents metabolic slowdown and makes it more likely that you will eat your way to success.

How frequent eating affects weight-loss hormones

Hormones are chemicals released by the body to trigger various functions within the system, including weight control. There are many hormones involved in this process and they influence everything from how hungry you feel, to how much fat your body stores or releases. But of all the hormones involved, three of the most important are cortisol, insulin, and leptin — all of which can be positively affected by eating frequently.

Cortisol, the belly-boosting hormone

Cortisol is a stress hormone that is released if you leave too long between meals. It is released partly because "hunger" is stressful for your body, but also because cortisol is extremely good at breaking down muscle mass, so your body calls it up to help it create energy quickly. But cortisol is also good at shuttling the excess calories you consume into your fat stores — particularly those around your abdominal area. This isn't good for your waistline but more importantly it is also incredibly bad for your health. A higher percentage of intra-abdominal fat, as this is known, is one of the main predictors of an increased risk of heart disease. Eating frequent small meals will slash cortisol levels, because your body doesn't need to cry out for that emergency energy supply. Trials conducted by Dr David Jenkins at the University of Toronto found that eating mini meals throughout the day cut cortisol by 17 percent in just two weeks.

Insulin, the sugar-shuttling hormone

The same Toronto trial also found a dramatic drop in insulin levels in people eating little and often. Now to anyone who understands basic biology this might sound odd; insulin is produced when we eat to actively transfer the sugar created from food into our muscle or, in the case of any excess, into our fat stores (with the stomach area, again, being a particularly common dumping ground). By cutting cortisol, you also cut insulin production as the two work together, but more basically, the amount of insulin produced if you eat a moderate meal or a light snack is far less than that released after the larger meals you consume on other eating plans. This limits the level of insulin in the body as a whole, which is positive since exposure to regularly high levels of insulin makes cells less responsive to it.

Leptin, the anti-hunger hormone

Finally, eating little and often also triggers the regular release of the hormone leptin, which is an appetite suppressant. It is released after eating and its concentration in the body decreases the longer you go without food. By eating little but more frequently, you regularly trigger leptin release, which means that you don't just feel less hungry because you are taking in regular food, but you are also increasing the production of the hormone that prevents overeating. According to scientists at the University of the Witwatersrand in South Africa, dieters naturally consume 27 percent less calories when eating the little-and-often way than they do when asked to consume three square meals, but they don't feel hungry while they are doing it and neither will you.

Could frequent eating cure your food addiction?

The final chemical controlled by eating little and often is neuropeptide Y (NPY). This isn't strictly a hormone, but a protein that stimulates cravings for carbohydrates. Oddly, if you get too hungry and then eat carbohydrate-based foods, instead of the levels of NPY going down, they actually increase causing you to binge, and your one-cookie treat turns into a diet-destroying four, five or more. This then starts to become a habit, causing you to crave those foods every time you get hungry, and before you know it your once-a-week candy bar has become a daily occurrence. By eating regularly, however, you never have an empty stomach and these cravings are kept in check before they can even start. For many people, this alone could be the key to ultimate weight loss.

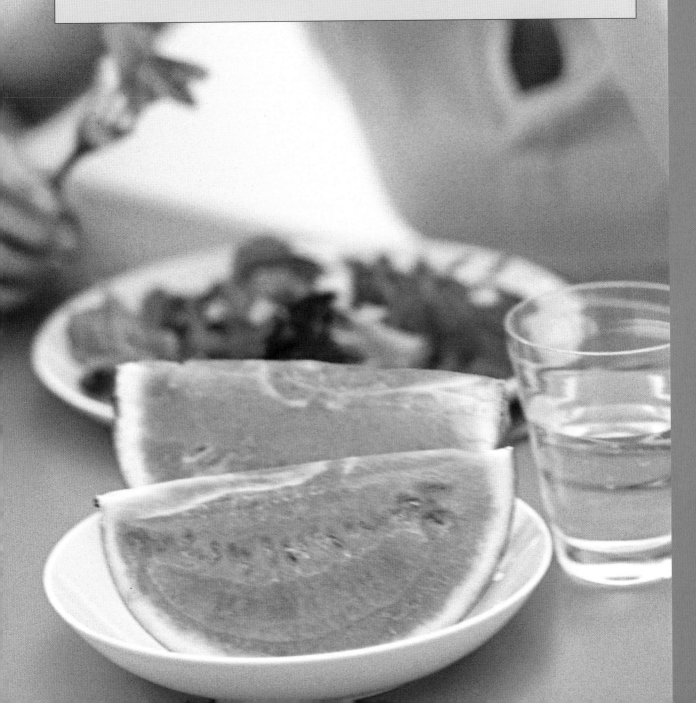

What this diet does to your weight

While the effects of this frequent-eating plan can be measured from head to toe, its effects on your waistline are the most compelling aspect, particularly the question of how much weight you can lose and how quickly you can eliminate it.

On this plan the average 143 lb woman will lose around $2^1/_4$ lb a week. If you weigh more than this (male or female), you will lose a little more, particularly in the first two weeks when weight loss is generally more rapid. Overall most people who stick to the guidelines will be at least 8–14 lb lighter after six weeks.

In a world where some diets promise weight loss of 14 lb in two weeks or less, that may sound a little slow, but remember you will be losing weight with no hunger pangs and, as you'll discover on pages 18–19, you will be doing it by eating the foods you want rather than forcing down foods that you don't like. You'll also be dieting without cutting any major food group (and therefore won't suffer the intense cravings for banned food that

you'd develop otherwise). By eating more frequently, you will also ensure that the maximum percentage possible of this weight loss is fat, not lean, metabolically active muscle, making it more likely that you'll keep that weight off once the diet is over.

It is also possible that weight comes off your stomach faster than many other parts of your body because your insulin levels are lowered. While it is true that it is impossible to lose weight from one specific part of the body simply by cutting calories, it has been shown that diets that control insulin do tend to promote rapid weight loss from the abdominal area; because this diet also lowers levels of the hormone cortisol, the weight-loss effect could be even greater.

Finally, there is one more way that eating the little-and-often way can change your weight — by giving you the energy to make exercise part of your life. Within two or three days of eating this way you will notice your energy levels soar. This happens because regular eating balances blood-sugar levels, preventing the sudden rises and falls that are a common cause of daytime fatigue. No wonder therefore that trials at Queen Margaret University College in Belfast discovered that those eating more frequently are far more likely to exercise than those eating three square meals a day. You will find simple exercise suggestions on pages 27, 43, 51, and 90 of the plan but should your new-found energy make you feel like even more exertion, then you can add three to five workouts of at least 30 minutes a week. Good exercises to choose are jogging, cycling, swimming, aerobics classes, or sports like tennis and badminton.

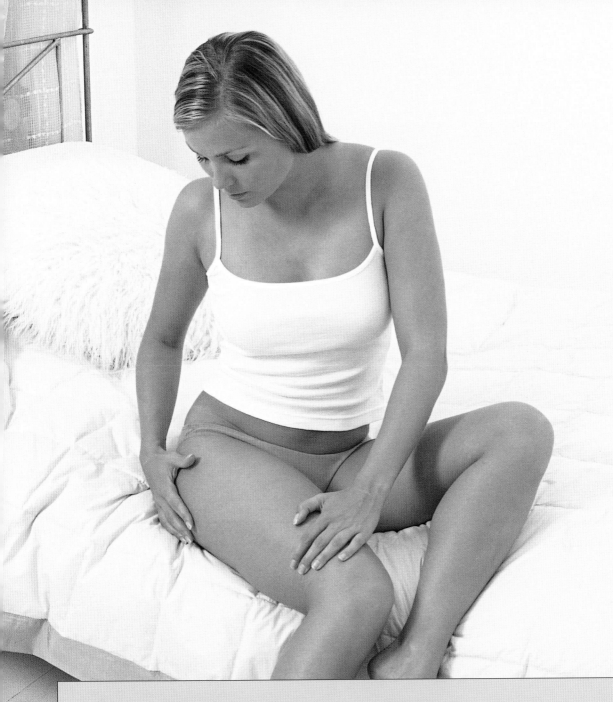

Do you need to alter your calorie-intake on this plan?

The meals and snacks suggested as part of this plan add up to around 1500 calories a day. For anyone who weighs 120–182 lb, you don't need to change anything. If you weigh over 182 lb this number of calories is a little too low; to prevent your metabolism slowing down and to avoid hunger pangs you should add another 200 calories a day by doubling the size of your morning and afternoon snacks. If you weigh less than 120 lb, you will need to cut calories by reducing portions in your main meals. But before you consider cutting calories, please do this simple calculation: divide your weight in kilograms by your height in meters squared. If you score under 18.5 using this calculation, you are already underweight for your height and really shouldn't try to lose any more weight.

What else does this diet do for you?

Weight loss isn't the only positive benefit of eating little and often. Because it influences levels of so many important hormones in the body, this eating plan has been proven to create positive health benefits from top to toe. By eating this way you could:

• **Lower your cholesterol** People who eat frequent meals have five percent less cholesterol in their system than those eating just one or two large meals a day according to researchers at the Institute of Public Health in Cambridge, UK.

• **Reduce the risk of atherosclerosis** In trials at London's Charing Cross Hospital, smokers eating little and often had 50 percent less risk of developing harmful plaque deposits on their arteries than those eating three square meals a day.

• **Cut the risk of diabetes** Type II diabetes occurs when the body becomes resistant to the amount of insulin flooding the system. By lowering insulin levels you

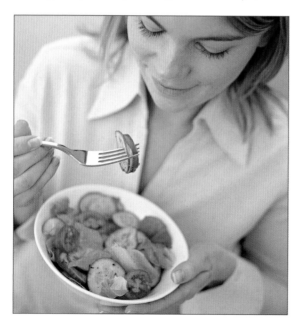

reduce the risk of this happening and therefore reduce the risk of diabetes.

• **Eat a greater variety of nutrients** Frequent eaters have higher levels of vitamin C and other nutrients in their systems, according to research at Queen Margaret University College in Belfast. It has also been found that people who eat little and often consume lower levels of fat and tend to eat more fruit and vegetables than less frequent eaters.

• **Fewer colds and flu** People who take in high levels of vitamin C report fewer sick days than other eaters. When you eat, it raises the levels of an immunity-boosting substance called *gamma interferon*, which means that eating little and often could also potentially influence the strength of your immune system.

• **Fight PMS** The British-based Women's Nutritional Advisory Service recommends eating little and often as a primary part of its groundbreaking PMS treatment plan. This works by regulating the low blood-sugar levels that are a major contributor to PMS symptoms. Eating regularly is also part of the treatment plan for other hormonal problems like polycystic ovary syndrome.

• **Reduce the risk of premature labor** While no one suggests that pregnant women should attempt to lose weight, organizing your recommended daily calories into a little-and-often eating plan seems to cut the risk of premature birth, according to research by the University of North Carolina.

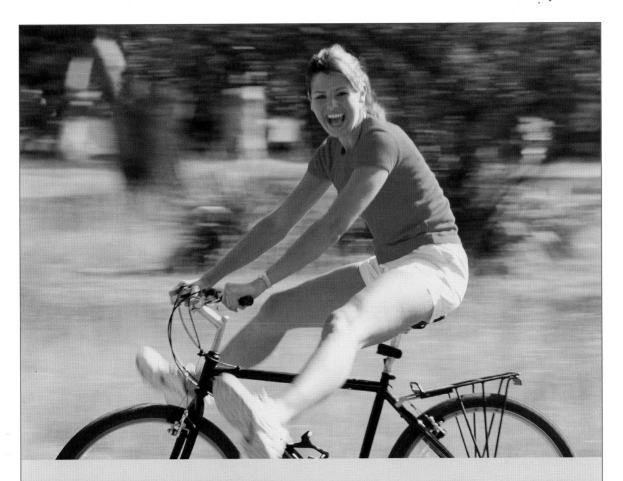

Five groups who will love the plan

While anybody can lose weight on this little-and-often plan, there are some groups of people who will particularly benefit:

• **Yo yo dieters** Because you may have lost muscle mass in the past, your metabolic rate may already be lower than it should be. This plan will stop things getting worse. If you exercise more than normal you could actually increase muscle mass.

• **Older dieters** Not only does appetite diminish as you get older, which makes large meals unappealing and unpalatable, research published in the *American Journal of Clinical Nutrition* states that the over-60s actually don't metabolize large meals as well as younger eaters, increasing the chance that the calories they consume will be stored as fat.

• **People with big appetites** If you normally quit diets because you are hungry, this is the diet for you — you will feel constantly satisfied. To boost that feeling of fullness, choose snacks containing proteins such as meat, fish, dairy, nuts, or seeds, which are more filling than those based purely on carbohydrates.

• **Tired types** You will notice an increase in energy levels within two or three days on this plan; you will be less likely to get sidetracked by sugary snacks designed to boost your energy.

• **Exercisers** Some low-calorie plans make exercise feel incredibly difficult because you just don't have the energy to work out. Because this plan lets you eat frequently, it is far easier to give yourself an injection of energy before your workout and refuel afterwards.

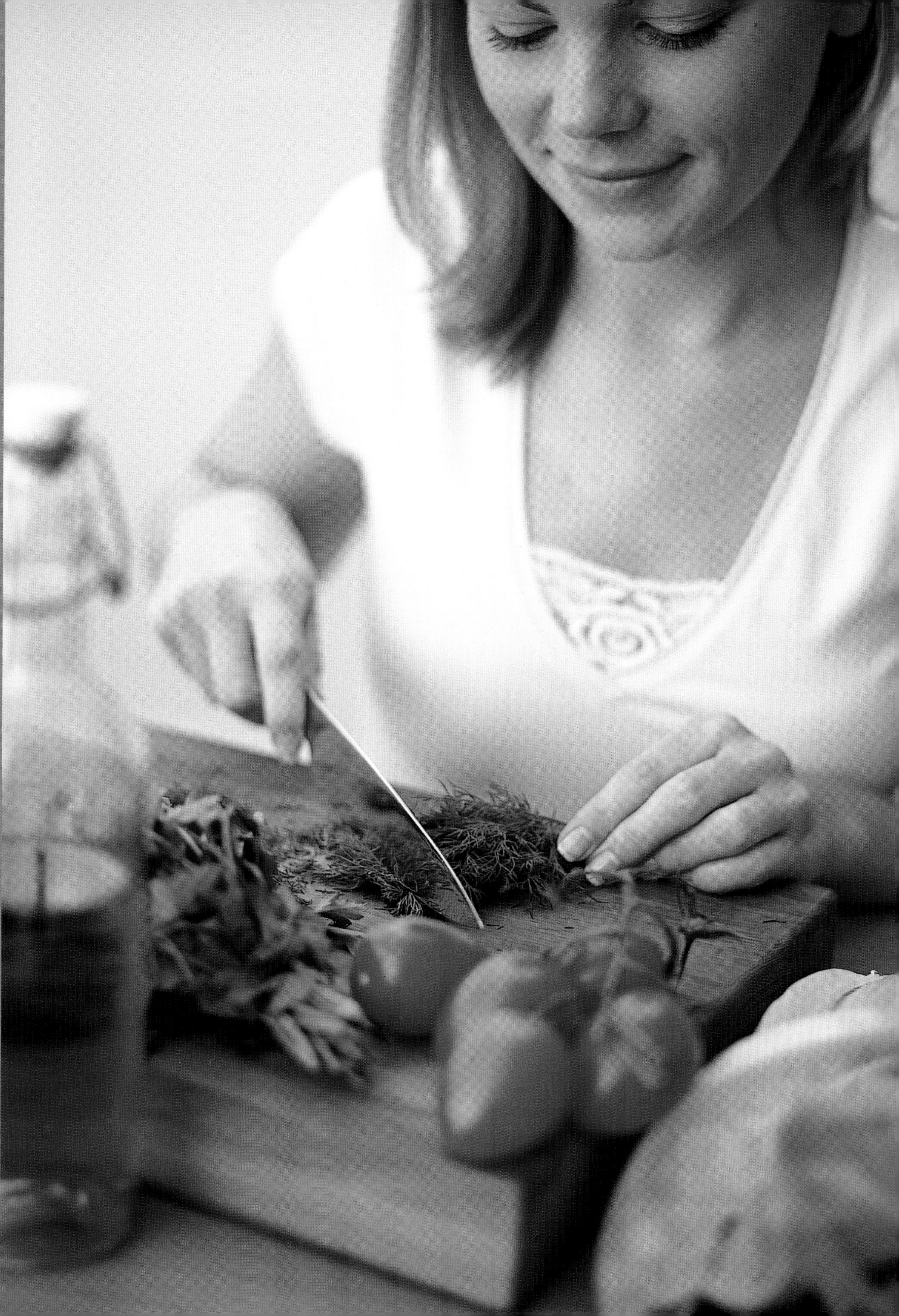

What to eat and when to eat it

You already know that you are going to be eating six times a day on this plan, but as yet you have no idea what you can eat. That's because it's up to you. On this diet you choose exactly what's going to appear on your plate each day.

The reasoning behind this is simple — most dieters quit plans because the diets include foods they either don't like or can't fit into their lifestyle. Can you imagine the misery involved in trying to follow a diet plan set by someone who doesn't know your schedule, your budget, or your nutritional likes or dislikes for six meals a day?

On this little-and-often eating plan you effectively design your own diet from the 200-plus suggested meals featured on pages 22–121. All you need do is choose one breakfast, lunch, and dinner and three snacks each day. And if you don't find anything there that suits you on any given day, you'll find guidelines on pages 124–125 that allow you to devise a plan that's totally personal to you. The result is that this diet becomes one you can follow no matter how many regimes you've quit in the past.

Ideally, you are aiming to space out your meals and snacks with a gap of roughly two to three hours between each meal and snack. The gap between meals and snacks should get smaller as the day progresses as it has been shown that you get hungry more frequently as the day goes on. Suggested times to eat are shown on the Eating Clock below, but you can adjust the times to suit your lifestyle.

You should, however, aim to eat your breakfast no later than one hour after you've woken up, because overnight your glycogen levels (the sugar you use as fuel) fall. It is believed that your body actually does a glycogen audit shortly after waking and what it finds determines the level of hunger you're going to feel throughout the day. If you refuel your glycogen levels early on in the day, your body will decide you don't need as much to eat today and as a result you'll feel less hungry. This will make your plan considerably easier to follow and keep any hunger pangs at bay.

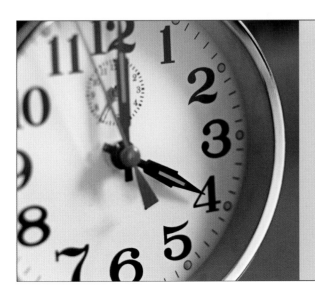

The Eating Clock

Here is an example of how your meals could be spaced out throughout your day.

7 a.m.	Breakfast
10 a.m.	Morning snack
1 p.m.	Lunch
4 p.m.	Afternoon snack
6.30 p.m.	Evening meal
9 p.m.	Evening snack

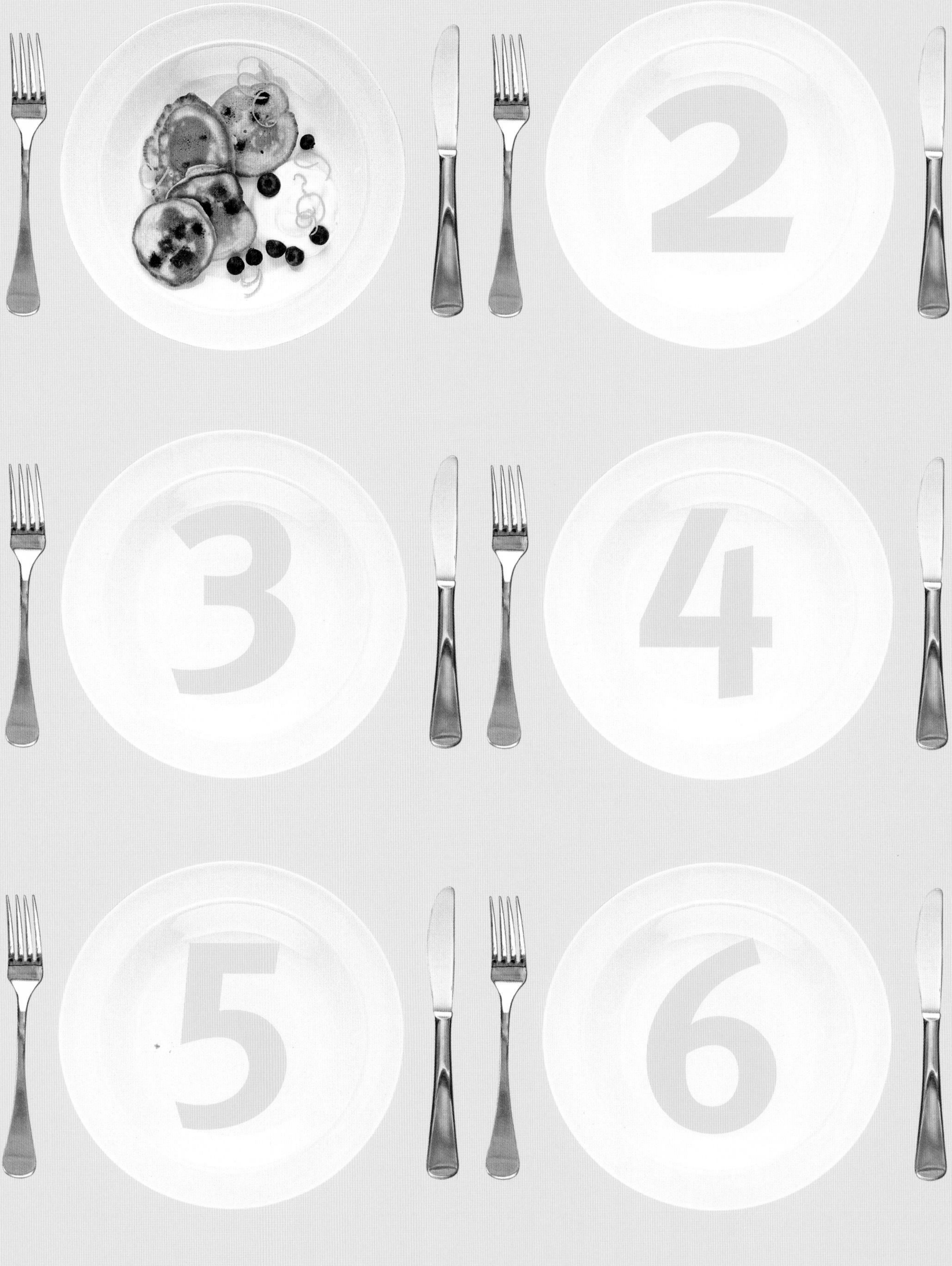
2
3
4
5
6

Breakfast

Breakfast is considered the most important meal of the day. Breakfast eaters generally take in more nutrients, less fat, and more fiber than breakfast skippers, which means they also tend to be healthier and more energized than those who don't eat first thing.

In fact, breakfast is so important that leading health researchers Belloc and Breslow named eating it as one of the "Seven Habits for Longevity" in their groundbreaking 1970s research. Eating breakfast is right up there with not smoking and exercising regularly in helping you live a long, disease-free life.

However, it is in the field of weight loss that breakfast truly shines. Breakfast eaters are 4.5 times less likely to be overweight than skippers, and weigh an average of 8 lb less overall. There are many reasons why this happens; breakfast reverses the metabolic slowdown that occurs while we sleep. Reversing this decline alone can increase your potential weight loss by just over $2^1/_4$ lb in a year. Many traditional breakfast foods also have weight-loss fighting powers of their own (see pages 26–27 for more details), while the simple act of eating first thing also triggers the body to produce optimum levels of the appetite-suppressing hormone leptin, high levels of which were found to be a major determinant of weight-loss success in trials held at the Western Human Nutrition Research Center in Davis, California. Researchers at the University of El Paso in Texas have discovered that calories eaten first thing actually seem to be more filling than the same number of calories eaten later in the day, which means that breakfast eaters actually consume less calories overall than those who think they are saving calories by skipping it.

But to get these positive effects you need to eat the right kind of breakfast. Many of the foods we eat first thing (including white toast, sugary cereals, and instant oatmeal) are high GI foods that convert very rapidly to sugar in the body. This causes blood-sugar levels to surge, then crash, and this crash triggers hunger pangs. Get your combinations right by filling your breakfasts with low glycemic carbohydrates (like multigrain breads, rolled oats, and bran cereals) or through including a little protein which slows digestion, and you will avoid this sugar seesaw and the extra calories you consume because of it.

Choose from 50 breakfasts

Each of these breakfasts combines the perfect mix of carbohydrates and proteins to rev up your metabolism and satisfy your appetite. They all contain at least one serving of fruit or vegetables to help you reach the recommended five or more a day. In terms of energy each breakfast provides around 250 calories (1050 kj); remember, calories eaten at this time of the day are particularly satisfying so it's okay to start with a relatively low-calorie meal.

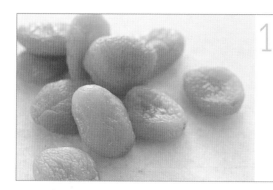

1 Five ready-to-eat **dried apricots**, chopped and mixed with 1 palmful of almonds. Add to a small carton of low-fat fromage frais or plain yogurt.

2 Small carton of low-fat **yogurt** topped with a sliced banana and 3 tablespoons of low-sugar granola.

3 $^2/_3$ cup **grapefruit juice**. Follow with 2 Melba toasts each topped with 2 tablespoons low-fat cream cheese.

4 $^1/_2$ cup **rolled oats** made with water and add 1 teaspoon of honey and 3 handfuls of any berry.

5 One **plain croissant** (around 2 oz) served with 2 handfuls of strawberries.

6 Two slices of **fruit loaf** topped with a scraping of low-fat spread and 1 fresh peach or pear or 7 oz canned peaches or pears in their natural juice.

7 Three **bacon slices**, with all fat removed, broiled then served with 1 egg scrambled and 4 mushrooms chopped and broiled.

FIVE HEALTH BENEFITS OF BREAKFAST

Weight loss isn't the only positive effect of eating breakfast — studies reveal it can affect our body in all manner of health-promoting ways:

Increased energy Researchers at Cardiff University, Wales found breakfast eaters have ten percent more energy than breakfast skippers, probably because the fiber in many breakfast foods helps fight constipation, a known cause of fatigue.

Healthier hearts Skipping breakfast increases levels of cholesterol in the body say researchers at the University of Nottingham in the UK. Exactly why isn't known.

Lowered diabetes risk Exposure to high levels of insulin in the body is one of the risk factors of type II diabetes, but the same Nottingham study found that breakfast eaters are more sensitive to the insulin produced in their body which naturally keeps levels lowered.

Fewer colds and flu When researchers in Cardiff looked at sickness rates, breakfast skippers generally experienced at least one minor illness in the ten-week study while eaters escaped.

Denser bones The higher levels of nutrients in the diets of breakfast eaters mean they tend to have thicker bones than skippers, reducing their risk of osteoporosis.

8 One low-fat **granola bar** with 1 chopped apple or pear and 1 cup low-fat or soy milk.

9 One serving of **Dried Fruit Compote** (see recipe on page 31) topped with 2 tablespoons of any flavor of low-fat yogurt or fromage frais.

10 One **egg** scrambled and served with 7 oz low-sugar baked beans.

11 One **fruit biscuit** (around 2 oz) topped with 1 teaspoon of low-sugar jelly. Accompany with 1 apple, pear, or any other piece of fruit.

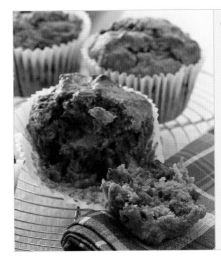

12 One **Apple and Blackberry Muffin** (see recipe on page 28) followed by half a grapefruit sprinkled with a little sweetener or $2/3$ cup of unsweetened grapefruit juice.

13 $1/3$ cup of any **cereal** (bran or corn flakes) topped with $2/3$ cup skim milk. Add 3 handfuls of any berry (fresh or frozen) and 6 almonds.

14 One slice of **multigrain toast** or thickly sliced bread topped with 1 sliced tomato, 1 slice of ham and 1 oz sliced mozzarella, eaten cold or broiled until the cheese starts to soften.

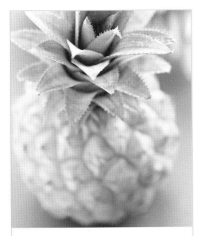

16 One slice of fresh **pineapple** or two slices canned in natural juice on half a bagel topped with 2 teaspoons of cream cheese. Accompany with $2/3$ cup tomato juice.

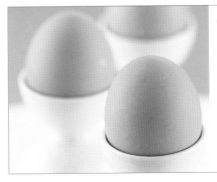

15 One **boiled egg** served with a slice of toast topped with a little yeast spread. Accompany with $2/3$ cup apple or other fruit juice.

17 Two slices of **toast** topped with 2 slices of processed cheese and 1 tomato sliced then broiled.

18 One small **bread roll** spread with a little ketchup or brown sauce and filled with 1 low-fat meat or vegetarian sausage, broiled and sliced. Add 1 tomato slice or a few mushrooms, sliced and broiled.

19 One slice of **multigrain or rye toast** topped with 1 teaspoon of peanut butter. Serve with 2 small fruits such as plum, kiwi, or apricot and $2/3$ cup of skim milk.

20 $2/3$ cup **Swiss-style muesli** made as directed with $2/3$ cup skim milk, soy milk, or water.

BEAT THE BREAKFAST EXCUSES

Many people can't face eating in the morning because they have no appetite. Strangely, skipping breakfast could be the reason behind this. Calories eaten first thing in the morning are incredibly filling, cutting down the amount we eat later in the day — skip breakfast, however, and you're more more likely to overeat at night sapping your appetite in the morning. Starting a breakfast habit will regulate your appetite and after two or three days of eating something light in the morning, food first thing will seem more appealing. Good breakfasts to start with are fruit salads, smoothies, or muesli bars that won't leave you feeling bloated.

Lack of time is another reason why people skip breakfast. Forget fiddly foods you need to cook or soak and choose breakfasts you can eat on the run like the Sticky Fruit and Nut Bars on page 34. These will keep for up to five days in the refrigerator, which means that you can make a batch at the weekend and simply grab one each day. Other good choices are rice cakes with peanut butter and fruit, fruit biscuits with jelly or a store-bought muesli bar with fruit and a glass of milk.

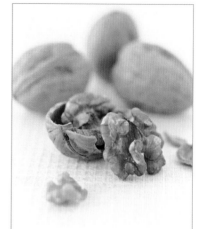

21 A small handful (around 1 oz) of **walnut halves**, 2 slices of lean ham, 2 slices of processed cheese, 1 sliced apple.

22 One small **pita bread** (about 4 inches in diameter) spread with 2 teaspoons of low-sugar jelly and 2 tablespoons low-fat cream cheese and filled with 1 peach sliced.

23 Two **wheat biscuit cereal** (or similar style cereal) topped with $2/3$ cup skim or soy milk. Top with 1 sliced pear, peach, or apple.

24 Four **rye crackers** topped with $1/4$ cup ricotta and 2 teaspoons of low-sugar jelly. Serve with 3 slices of pineapple or half a mango.

25 One **sweet waffle** topped with 4 oz fresh or canned cherries and 1 tablespoon of low-fat fromage frais or plain yogurt.

27 $1/2$ cup **low-sugar granola** topped with $2/3$ cup skim milk and 2 sliced strawberries.

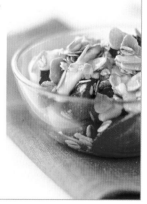

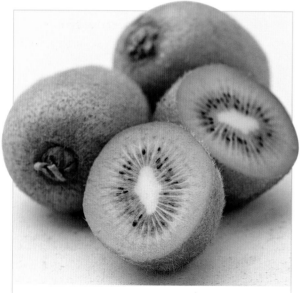

26 **Tropical fruit plate** of half a mango, 2 kiwifruit and 1 banana, all sliced and topped with 2 oz low-fat cottage cheese.

28 One serving of **Easy Corned Beef Hash** (see recipe on page 39) served with 2 broiled tomatoes.

29 One **crumpet** topped with a teaspoon of honey, served with 1 cup skim milk made into a smoothie with 2 handfuls of berries.

30 One serving of **Fruit Salad** (see recipe on page 35).

31 One **egg** scrambled and mixed with 1 1/2 oz smoked salmon slices chopped into small pieces. Serve on 1 slice of multigrain toast.

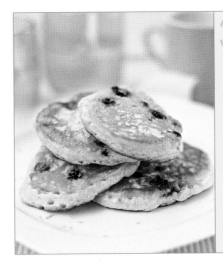

32 One serving of **Blueberry and Lemon Pancakes** (see recipe on page 32) topped with 1 tablespoon of low-fat fromage frais or low-fat plain or fruit-flavored yogurt.

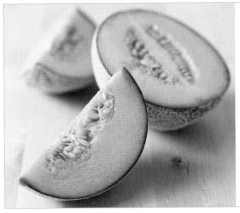

33 Half a **cantaloupe melon** topped with 3 handfuls of raspberries plus a 1 oz shredded wheat-type cereal biscuit topped with 2/3 cup skim milk.

34 **French toast** made from 1 slice of bread soaked in a mix of 1 egg and a little skim milk, then fried in a little oil spray. Serve with 1 sliced tomato or 2 handfuls of berries.

35 One serving of **Creamy Mushrooms on Toast** (see recipe on page 30).

36 Small carton of **low-fat yogurt** topped with a small handful (about 1 oz) of pumpkin seeds and 1 sliced nectarine or other fruit.

37 1/3 cup **quinoa** made into porridge with 2/3 cup skim milk and 2/3 cup water. Add a pinch of salt and/or sugar to taste. Top with a sliced persimmon, peach, or pear.

38 One **poached egg** served on a bed of unlimited wilted spinach and topped with 1 slice of ham and 1 tablespoon of hollandaise sauce.

QUICK QUESTION

A lot of the breakfasts recommended here include eggs which I thought raised cholesterol — how many eggs a week is it safe to eat?

Eggs have been unfairly demonized; the current thinking is that they don't play a significant part in raising cholesterol. By cutting them out of your diet, you are eliminating a vital source of protein and reducing your intake of many vital vitamins. Eggs are a major source of the antioxidant lutein, which helps protect eyesight from UV damage. The latest advice is one or two eggs a day if you don't have a cholesterol problem, and if you do have cholesterol problems, two or three eggs a week.

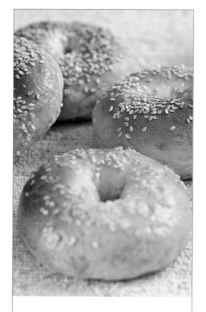

39 Half a **bagel** topped with 2 bacon slices and 1 sliced tomato, both broiled.

THE BEST DIET-BOOSTING BREAKFAST FOODS

While eating breakfast will help your weight loss, many of the foods we commonly eat first thing can actually boost your dieting effects. The four most powerful are:

Grapefruit This reduces the body's sensitivity to the fat-storage hormone insulin, potentially lowering levels of this within the body. In trials at Scripps Research Institute in San Diego, people lost 10 lb in three months simply by adding grapefruit or its juice before their meals.

Milk and dairy products Research from the University of Tennessee has found that these help promote the body's fat-burning process by actually turning fat-storing cells into fat-burning ones.

Breakfast cereals Packed with fiber (which actually binds to fat molecules in the body, reducing the amount you absorb), breakfast cereals are also a good source of iron, a mineral vital for healthy metabolism.

Eggs Studies at the University of Rochester in the US found that people who eat eggs for breakfast eat less calories on that day and the day after. It is believed eggs contain a type of protein that is particularly filling.

40 Two **apples or pears**, halved and spread with 1 teaspoon each of chocolate spread or peanut butter. Serve with ²/₃ cup of skim milk.

41 4 oz **prunes** canned in natural juice topped with a small carton of low-fat Greek or plain yogurt, 1 teaspoon of honey, and a sprinkle of low-sugar granola or pumpkin seeds.

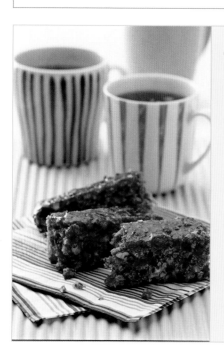

42 One **Sticky Fruit and Nut Bar** (see recipe on page 34) accompanied by a cup of black coffee, tea with a little skim milk, or some green tea. If you normally take sugar, switch to sweetener.

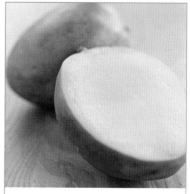

43 **Smoothie** made from 2 apricots, half a mango and 1 peach mixed with 1 cup skim milk and 1 oz soft tofu.

44 **Whey protein shake** (2 scoops mixed with ²/₃ cup skim milk and ¹/₃ cup water) with 2 rye crispbreads topped with 2 teaspoons of low-sugar jelly. Serve with 1 orange, peach, or similar fruit.

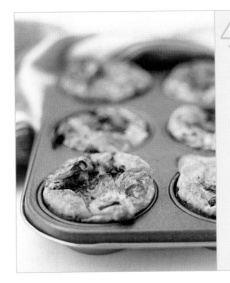

45 Three **Broccoli and Spinach Eggahs** (see recipe on page 36) served with 1 tablespoon of low-sugar baked beans, any piece of fruit, or ²/₃ cup of any unsweetened fruit juice.

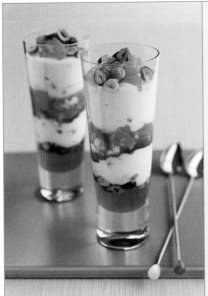

46 One serving of **Nutty Passionfruit Yogurt** (see recipe on page 38) — if you don't eat nuts it's okay to leave them out of the recipe, or you can replace them with an equivalent quantity of pumpkin, sunflower, or hemp seeds.

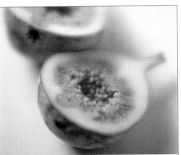

47 Three **fresh figs**, sliced and topped with 1 tablespoon each of low-fat plain yogurt. Sprinkle each with 1 teaspoon of sunflower or pumpkin seeds.

DIET POWER-UP

If you can get out for a 30-minute walk at breakfast time you will increase your weight loss by at least ¹/₃ lb a week, plus by walking on an empty stomach you will increase the amount of fat you burn, potentially leading to faster inch-loss as well. It's not recommended that you do more intensive exercise on an empty stomach; have something light such as a piece of fruit or toast before you start. And remember to eat your breakfast as soon as you get back home to prevent low glycogen stores making you feel hungry.

48 One slice of **multigrain or rye toast** topped with 5 oz low-sugar baked beans.

49 Three **rice cakes or oatcakes** topped with half a teaspoon of peanut butter each and slices of 1 apple.

50 One serving of **Easy Corned Beef Hash** (see recipe on page 39).

Breakfast recipes

The following recipes are all quick and easy ways to liven up your morning eating choices. Some are the perfect treat for a weekend breakfast while others are quick for busy mornings throughout the rest of the week. All the recipes are so tasty you will forget that you're dieting.

Apple and blackberry muffins

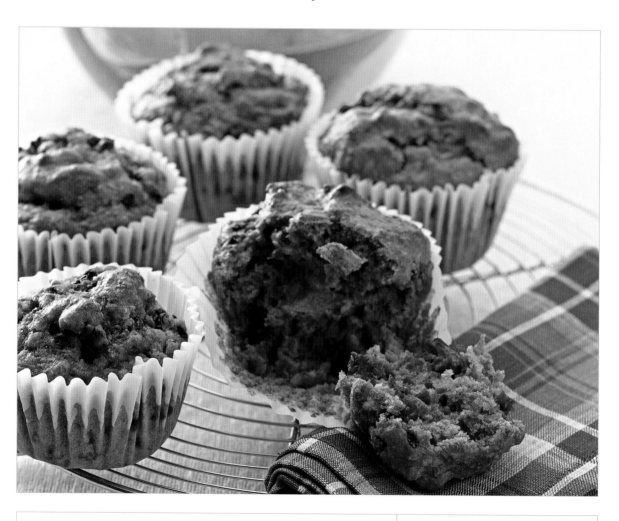

Makes 12
Preparation time 15 minutes
Cooking time 20–30 minutes

Nutritional values
Calories 203
Kilojoules 854
Protein 4 g
Carbohydrates 22 g
Fat 11 g

6 tablespoons light brown sugar

1 red apple, about 5 oz, cored and diced

1¹/₂ cups blackberries, roughly chopped

1 teaspoon ground cinnamon

2 cups all-purpose wholewheat flour

4 teaspoons baking powder

2 eggs, beaten

¹/₂ cup low-fat milk

¹/₂ cup canola oil, plus extra for cooking

1 Mix together the sugar, diced apple, blackberries, and ground cinnamon.

2 Sift the flour and baking powder into a bowl and make a well in the center. In a separate bowl mix together the eggs, milk, and oil.

3 Pour the liquid into the middle of the flour and stir until blended. Stir in the fruit mixture, taking care not to over-mix.

4 Divide the mixture among the sections of a 12-hole muffin pan, lightly oiled or lined with paper cups, and bake in a preheated oven, 400°F, for 20–30 minutes or until a tester inserted into the center comes out clean. Transfer the muffins to a wire rack to cool. The muffins can be stored in an airtight container for up to 3 days.

Canola oil

Canola oil may not be something you've used before but it can be a good addition to the pantry. Known in the UK as rapeseed oil, it comes from the seeds of bright yellow rapeseed flowers. It has quite a mild taste so it is great for recipes such as muffins, cakes, and other desserts that might be overpowered by a heavy oil. Canola is also a mono-unsaturated oil (like olive oil), high in vitamin E and healthy omega-3 fats. It shouldn't be the only oil in your cupboard as it does contain transfats, but in recipes such as this, canola oil is a great choice.

Measuring your results

Morning isn't just the best time to power up your weight loss — it is also the most accurate time to monitor it. Weigh yourself first thing in the morning after you've been to the bathroom and before you eat your breakfast. It is best to do it just once a week, but always on the same day of the week since variables such as how much exercise you did the day before, how much fluid you drank, and what foods you consumed can all make a difference to how much fluid you retain in a day; while these factors differ from day to day, very often you'll practice the same behaviors on the same days of the week.

Creamy mushrooms on toast

4 slices of wholewheat bread

1 tablespoon avocado oil

1 tablespoon lime juice

1 small onion, chopped

8 mushrooms, sliced

1 tablespoon light soy sauce

2 tablespoons ricotta cheese

1 Place the bread on a cookie sheet and bake in a preheated oven, 350°F, for 5 minutes.

2 Meanwhile, heat the oil in a skillet, add the lime juice and fry the onion and mushrooms until soft. Stir in the soy sauce followed by the ricotta.

3 Pour the mixture on top of the toasted wholewheat bread and serve immediately.

The best way to start the day?

For many people the day doesn't begin until they've had a cup of coffee, but is it really the healthiest choice? Well, it is not a bad thing. Recent studies have linked moderate caffeine consumption to a decreased risk of Parkinson's disease, liver cancer, and gallstones, and there is no truth to the rumor that the odd cup increases blood pressure. You shouldn't have more than three cups a day as the negative effects (like an increase in cortisol) have been found over this dose. This limit is also important if you are trying to lose weight, as too much coffee can cause blood-sugar crashes that trigger hunger pangs and sugar cravings.

This doesn't mean that you should limit other liquids on this little-and-often diet, as the more hydrated your body is the faster your metabolism runs. Aim for at least one cup of fluid with each meal or snack a day (plus two extra, perhaps as soon as you wake up and just before bed). These should be no-sugar drinks.

Serves 2
Preparation time 5 minutes
Cooking time 10 minutes

Nutritional values
Calories 207
Kilojoules 870
Protein 8 g
Carbohydrates 23 g
Fat 10 g

Dried fruit compote

1 lb mixed ready-to-eat dried fruit (such as apricots, figs, prunes, and cranberries)

1 cinnamon stick

1 star anise

2 cardamom pods

3/4 cup water

1/2 cup apple juice

low-fat plain yogurt, to serve

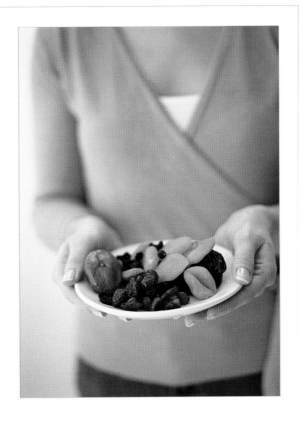

1 Place all the ingredients in a large saucepan and bring to a boil. Reduce the heat, cover, and simmer for 10 minutes.

2 Remove from the heat and set aside for at least 30 minutes so that the flavors can infuse. Serve warm with yogurt.

Serves 4
Preparation time 5 minutes, plus standing
Cooking time 10 minutes

Nutritional values
Calories 218
Kilojoules 930
Protein 4 g
Carbohydrates 51 g
Fat 1 g

Blueberry and lemon pancakes

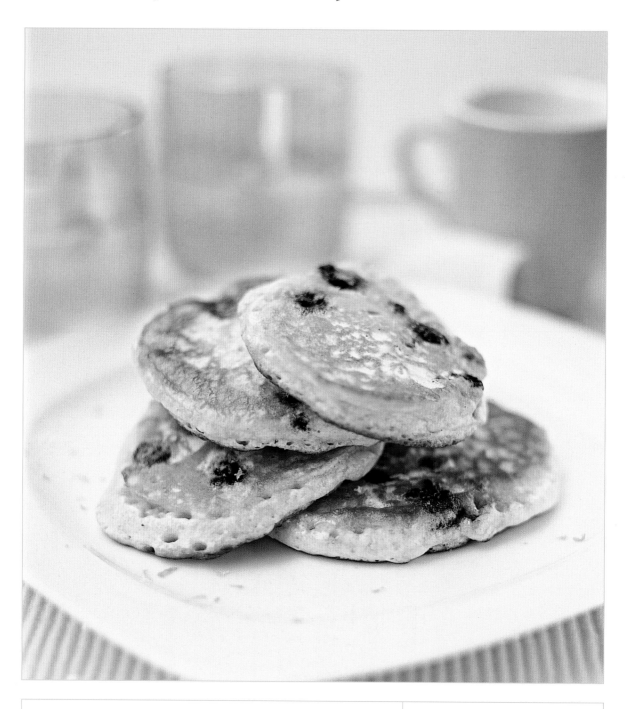

Serves 4
Preparation time 10 minutes
Cooking time 20 minutes

Nutritional values
Calories 197
Kilojoules 827
Protein 6 g
Carbohydrates 31 g
Fat 3 g

1 cup self-rising flour

1 teaspoon baking powder

finely grated zest of $^1/_2$ lemon

1 tablespoon superfine sugar

1 egg, lightly beaten

1 tablespoon lemon juice

$^2/_3$ cup low-fat milk

$^3/_4$ cup blueberries

vegetable oil, for frying

1 Sift the flour and baking powder into a bowl and stir in the lemon zest and sugar. Add the egg and lemon juice and gradually beat in the milk to make a smooth, thick batter. Stir in the blueberries.

2 Heat a griddle or large, nonstick skillet and rub it with a piece of paper towel drizzled with a little oil. Drop spoonfuls of the mixture, spaced well apart, on the griddle or pan and cook for 2–3 minutes until bubbles form on the surface and the underside is golden-brown.

3 Turn the pancakes over and cook the other side. Wrap them in a dish towel and keep hot while you cook the remaining mixture in the same way.

Superfood!

Blueberries were named as a major superfood by researchers at Tufts University in the US. Why? Not only are they the fresh fruit with the highest levels of antioxidants, blueberries seem to increase the levels of communication between nerve cells in the brain, which experts believe could help prevent age-related memory problems. Blueberries are high in ellagic acid, which helps fight cancer, and an ingredient called pterostilbine, which lowers cholesterol and protects our hearts. When eaten fresh, the only preparation that blueberries need is to be rinsed under a running tap. Try to include at least one serving a week in your diet.

Beware salt and sugar

Although many breakfast foods are healthy, salt is a common addition to many cereals while a lot of healthy-looking foods like yogurt can be very high in sugar. While the recommended intake of sugar is 40 g a day and the recommended intake of salt is 6 g (2.4 g sodium), this doesn't always mean much to us, so many experts suggest converting the grams in your foods to tablespoons to show how much you are really eating.

• For sugar, divide the number of grams of sugar on a label by 4.7 to give the amount in teaspoons and aim to eat no more than 8 $^1/_2$.

• For salt, every 1.9 grams of sodium is roughly 1 teaspoon of salt.

Sticky fruit and nut bars

$^1/_2$ cup all-purpose flour

1 cup pitted dates, roughly chopped

$^1/_4$ cup raw sugar

$^1/_2$ cup rolled oats

1 teaspoon baking powder

1 teaspoon ground cinnamon

$1^1/_3$ cups pecan nuts, roughly chopped

2 large eggs, lightly beaten

4 tablespoons canola oil

4 tablespoons reduced-sugar, rough-cut marmalade or apricot jelly

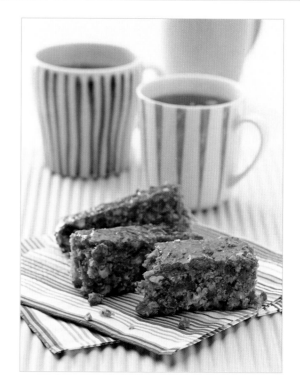

1 Sift the flour into a large bowl and mix in the remaining dry ingredients. Stir in the beaten eggs and oil and mix well.

2 Grease and line a 6 inch square pan. Pour the mixture into the pan, level the top and bake in a preheated oven, 350°F, for 30–35 minutes or until the top is firm. Allow to cool in the pan for 10 minutes then turn onto a wire rack.

3 Heat the marmalade or jelly in a small saucepan and brush it over the top of the cake. When it is cold, cut it into 12 bars. The bars can be stored in an airtight container for up to 5 days.

Makes 12
Preparation time 10 minutes
Cooking time 30–35 minutes

Nutritional values
Calories 230
Kilojoules 966
Protein 9 g
Carbohydrates 20 g
Fat 15 g

Fruit salad with banana cream

1 ruby grapefruit

2 oranges

2 kiwifruit, peeled

1 ripe banana

3/4 cup low-fat fromage frais or plain yogurt

1 tablespoon honey

1 Cut the top and bottom off the grapefruit with a serrated knife to reveal the flesh, then cut away the remaining peel and pith. Holding the fruit above a serving bowl, cut between the membranes to release the fruit segments. Repeat the process with the oranges.

2 Cut the kiwifruit in half, then into thin wedges. Mix with the citrus fruit. Cover and chill if making in advance.

3 Mash the banana with a fork and stir it into the fromage frais or yogurt with the honey. Spoon the fruit salad into bowls and serve topped with the banana cream.

Why eating breakfast may fight comfort eating

Many breakfast cereals and other wholegrains that make up an important part of our normal morning diets are incredibly high in the energy-giving B vitamins. All of these are important for mood regulation and for fighting the effects of stress — but thiamine (which is found in high doses in breakfast foods such as cereals, oats, egg yolks, and peanut butter) is particularly valuable for mood boosting. When researchers at the University of Wales, Swansea, asked women to include more sources of it in their diets they felt twice as happy in just two months. To add to the effects, try to eat your breakfast outside in fine weather, or at least in view of the window. Research from the University of British Columbia in Vancouver found that just 30 minutes of sunshine a day is enough to boost mood and prevent stress-induced snack attacks.

Serves 4
Preparation time 20 minutes

Nutritional values
Calories 164
Kilojoules 689
Protein 6 g
Carbohydrates 28 g
Fat 4 g

Broccoli and spinach eggahs

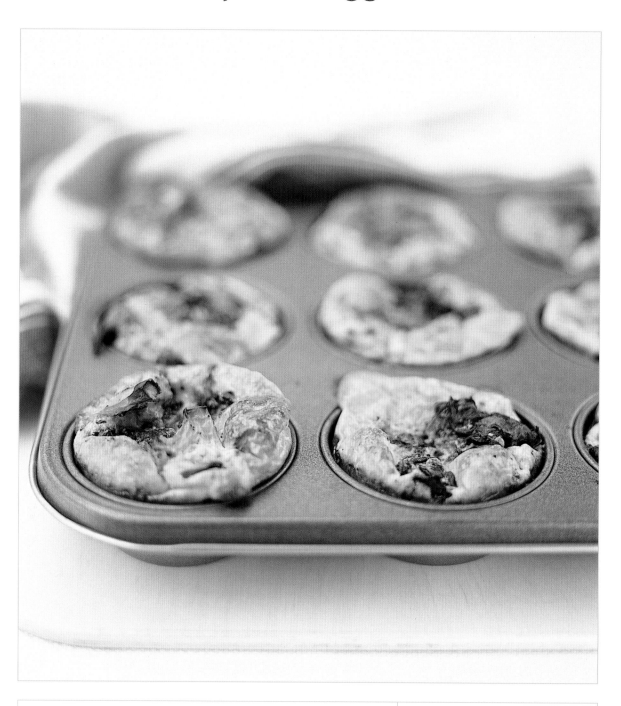

Makes 12
Preparation time 15 minutes
Cooking time 20 minutes

Nutritional values
Calories 72
Kilojoules 300
Protein 6 g
Carbohydrates 2 g
Fat 5 g

4 oz broccoli

3 cups young spinach leaves

6 eggs

1¹/₄ cups low-fat milk

2 tablespoons grated Parmesan cheese

large pinch of ground nutmeg

oil, for cooking

salt and pepper

1 Cut the broccoli into small florets and thickly slice the stems. Put in a steamer set over boiling water, cover, and cook for 3 minutes. Add the spinach and cook for 1 minute more or until the spinach has just wilted.

2 Beat the eggs, milk, Parmesan, nutmeg, and a little salt and pepper together in a pitcher.

3 Divide the broccoli and spinach among the sections of a deep, lightly oiled, 12-hole muffin pan and cover with the egg mixture. Bake in a preheated oven, 375°F, for about 15 minutes or until lightly browned, well risen, and the egg mixture has set. Leave in the pan for 1–2 minutes, then loosen the edges with a knife and turn out.

Brilliant brassicas

Broccoli may not seem like a standard breakfast food but it is so vital for health that anything that encourages us to eat it more often should be applauded. Broccoli and other members of the brassica family such as cauliflower, cabbage, and kale are known to be high sources of sulforaphane, which experts believe to be the most potent cancer-fighting chemicals discovered to date. Just 2–3 servings of broccoli a week is enough to reduce risk. If you don't like the slightly bitter taste of broccoli combining it with dairy products can disguise it.

The secret of diet success

Buy a scale. Not the ones that you stand on to monitor your progress, but the ones you use to measure the portion sizes of food — if there is one meal where this is absolutely vital it is breakfast, especially if you're a cereal fan. Research from the University of Illinois has discovered that when we serve ourselves food from a large package we tend to dish out up to 36 percent more than we would if we served ourselves from a smaller pack. It will also help to buy a tall, narrow glass. When we drink out of a glass shaped like this, we feel satisfied with 76 percent less fluid than we do if we're drinking out of a short wide glass. This is good news as many drinks can be calorific but because they don't fill us up, we tend not to notice how much we're consuming.

Nutty passionfruit yogurts

2 passionfruit

1 cup low-fat plain yogurt

2 tablespoons honey

3 tablespoons hazelnuts, roughly chopped

4 clementines, peeled and chopped into
   small pieces

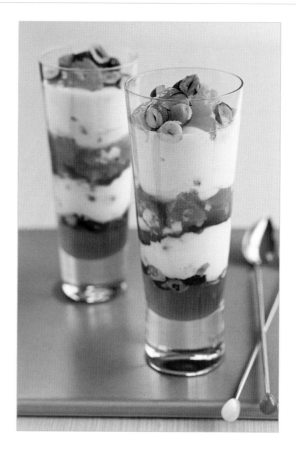

1 Halve the passionfruit and scoop the pulp into a
large bowl. Add the yogurt and mix together gently.

2 Put 1 tablespoonful of honey in the bottom of
each of 2 narrow glasses and sprinkle with a few
hazelnuts. Spoon half the yogurt over the nuts and
arrange half the clementine pieces on top.

3 Repeat the layering, finishing with a few
hazelnuts on the top of the dish. Keep chilled
until you are ready to eat.

Serves 2
Preparation time 5 minutes

Nutritional values
Calories 260
Kilojoules 1092
Protein 34 g
Carbohydrates 10 g
Fat 14 g

Easy corned beef hash

1 teaspoon vegetable oil

1 onion, roughly chopped

12 oz new potatoes, cooked and roughly chopped

10 oz corned beef, roughly chopped

1 tablespoon chopped parsley

Worcestershire sauce, to taste

pepper

1 Heat the oil in a large, nonstick skillet. Add the onion and fry for 5 minutes until softened. Add the potatoes and corned beef and continue to cook for 6–7 minutes, turning the mixture occasionally so that parts of it become crisp.

2 Add the parsley and stir through the mixture, season to taste with Worcestershire sauce and pepper and serve immediately.

Creating a healthy future

Next time you are tempted to skip breakfast, tell yourself that you're not just doing yourself good by eating it, you'll also be helping your kids, too. It's been proven that children who live in families where the adults are seen to eat and enjoy breakfast are more likely to develop the habit themselves. Kids will particularly enjoy the breakfast selections here, including bagels with cream cheese and pineapple, sweet waffles with fruit and yogurt, French toast, or boiled egg and toast.

Health booster

If you are starting your day with a bowl of cereal, make sure you don't leave any milk in the bottom of the bowl. Around 40 percent of the folic acid found in breakfast cereal is actually absorbed into the milk, and if you leave any you'll be missing out on this vital ingredient. Vegetarians pouring calcium-enriched soy milk over their cereal should also ensure that they shake the bottle or carton well before pouring as the calcium can settle at the bottom. Calcium is one of the most important fat-burning nutrients so far discovered.

Serves 4
Preparation time 10 minutes
Cooking time 11–12 minutes

Nutritional values
Calories 227
Kilojoules 953
Protein 22 g
Carbohydrates 17 g
Fat 7 g

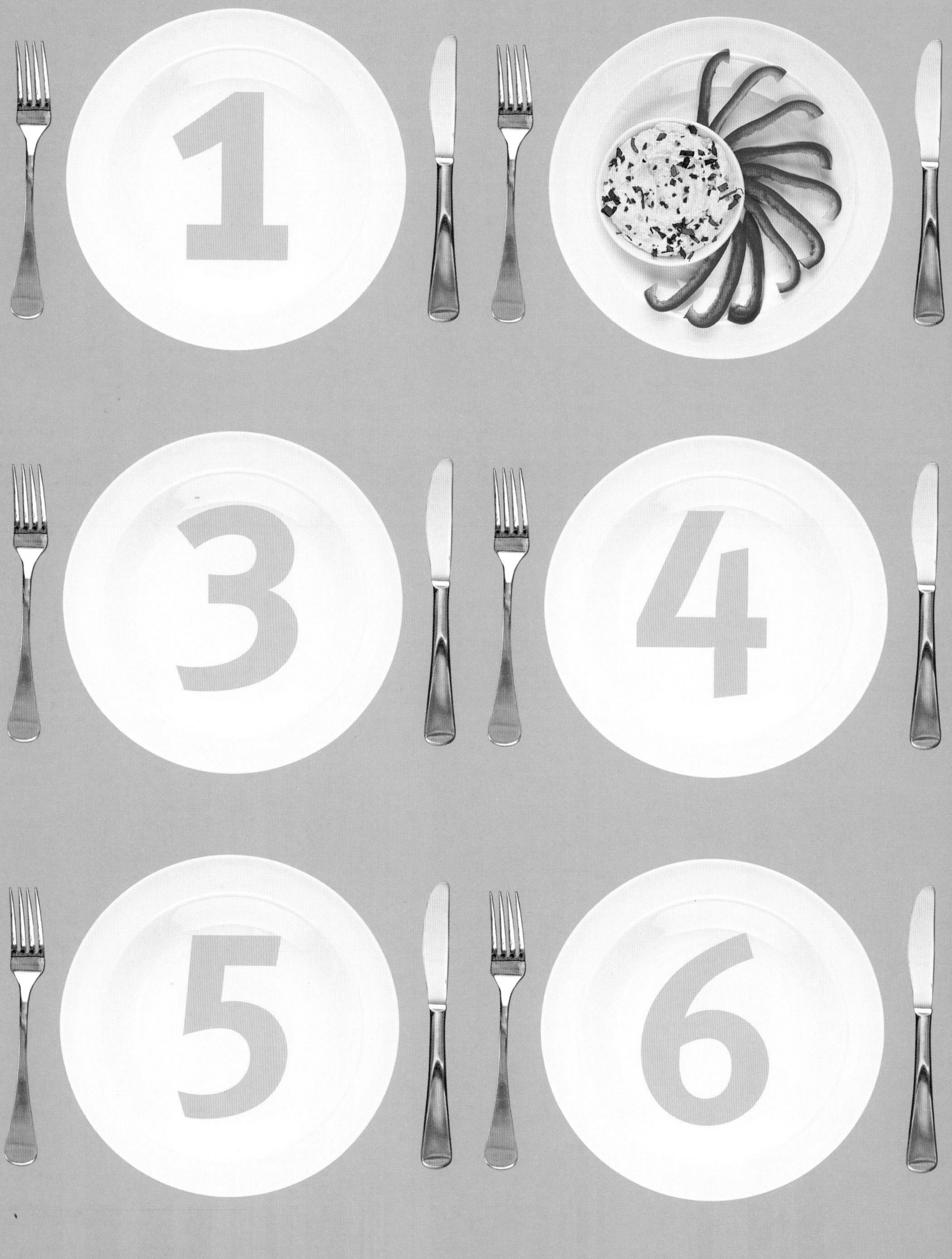

Mid-morning snack

When we hear the word snack we often think of sweet or salty treats, usually found in bright packages and gobbled while we're on the run. With your new eating regime of six meals a day, things are very different.

You will be eating lots of fruit, vegetables, nuts, seeds, and maybe a few foods you wouldn't think of snacking on, like fish and chicken. These foods give the body the highest metabolic boost of all. Remember, within 30 minutes of eating a meal high in protein (found in foods such as fish, chicken, meat, and dairy products) your metabolic rate can rev up as high as 30 percent for up to two hours. And when you eat a meal or snack high in fiber (contained in nuts, seeds, fruit, and vegetables) it revs up as much as 15 percent. This means you'll burn more calories than normal even if all you're doing physically is sitting at work making telephone calls or enjoying a weekend lounge with a good book.

Of all the meals you will eat on your six-meals-a-day plan, this may be the one that feels the most strange to integrate into your day. Most of us rarely snack mid-morning (unless we skipped breakfast), thinking that we should save our calories for lunch instead. We've already explained metabolically why this is a bad idea — if you are breakfasting at 7 a.m. and not eating lunch until 1 p.m. your body will have already used the calories you consumed and be crying out for fuel, potentially encouraging you to overeat at lunchtime. But by eating just a few bites of the right kind of snack midway through your morning, you will prevent both the metabolic slowdown and any diet-derailing hunger pangs.

But it doesn't matter how important mid-morning snacking is to your health, if the snacks require too much preparation you are not going to want to eat them. Because of this it is important to choose snacks that are portable and easy to nibble while you work. Over the page you will find 40 examples, all perfectly planned to give your body the optimum mid-morning boost.

Choose from 40 snacks

Each snack here contains around 100 calories, and is generally high in protein to create the optimum metabolic boost right from the start of the day. Most snacks are easily portable and can be kept in a package in your desk drawer for the week. Others are more elaborate, allowing you to treat yourself at weekends or on days when you want something a little more exotic than pumpkin seeds.

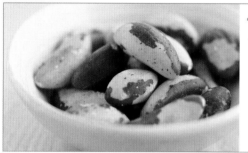

1 Six **Brazil nuts,** 3 whole shelled walnuts or 7–8 smaller nuts like almonds or hazelnuts.

2 One serving of **Bloody Marianna** (see recipe on page 48) served with 1 Melba toast spread with a little low-fat cream cheese.

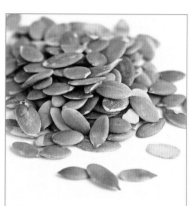

3 Three slices of **ham** served with 2 teaspoons of relish.

4 Three slices of **chicken** roll or sliced turkey served with 2 fresh apricots.

5 1 oz low-fat **edam cheese** served with 8–10 red grapes.

6 Three **falafel balls** with $1/4$ teaspoon of sweet chili sauce.

7 Two **rye crackers** topped with $1/6$ of an avocado, mashed.

8 One handful of **pumpkin** or sunflower seeds.

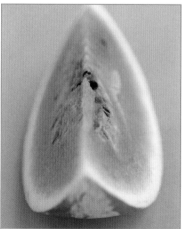

9 One slice of **watermelon** (about $1/8$ of a fruit), chopped and served with 1 oz feta cheese, also chopped into small chunks.

WARNING — HIGH-CALORIE SNACKS AHEAD

While foods such as nuts and seeds are far healthier snacks than savory snacks or chocolate, ounce for ounce, they actually have roughly the same amount of calories. So measure portions carefully, and ideally keep them well out of sight when it's not snack time.

According to research at the University of Illinois, people eat three times more of a snack food if they can see it from their desk than they do if it is hidden in a bottom drawer and six times more than if it is locked away. If, however, you really can't control yourself around nuts, seeds, rice cakes, or any other snack food, it might be best to switch to another option. While one handful of nuts might only contain 100 calories, if you have two or three it's not going to be good news for your diet.

DID YOU CLIMB ANY STAIRS TODAY?

Experts at the University of North Carolina in the US estimate that if we climbed just two flights of stairs each day (instead of taking the elevator at work or standing on the escalator in the shopping mall) we'd lose 6 lb a year without having to change anything at all about our diet.

While there is no fixed exercise stipulated on this frequent-eating diet, you can make it a rule to build in as much incidental activity as possible each day. Ideally, buy yourself a pedometer and aim for the recommended 10,000 steps a day; this will burn 500 extra calories and boost your weight loss by 1 lb a week.

Activities such as parking in the farthest car park, using the bathroom on the floor above your office, or even just standing up while you make phone calls (which burns roughly 30 percent more calories than sitting down), all add up to an increased level of weight loss.

10 A **protein shake** made from 2 scoops of protein powder mixed with 3/4 cup water.

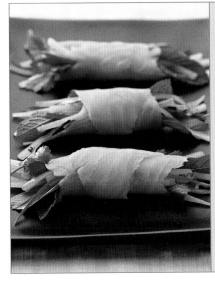

11 Three **Smoked Salmon Thai Rolls** (see recipe on page 46) or 1 1/4 oz of smoked salmon served with some slices of cucumber, celery, or red pepper.

12 Two **oatcakes** spread with 2 tablespoons low-fat cottage cheese and topped with 1 sliced kiwifruit.

13 Four small **sushi rolls** (vegetarian or fish such as shrimp or salmon — avoid fillings with mayonnaise).

14 One **Parmesan and Herb Scone** (see recipe on page 49).

15 Small carton of low-fat **cottage cheese** with pineapple.

16 Three slices of **salami** served with 4 sun-dried tomatoes.

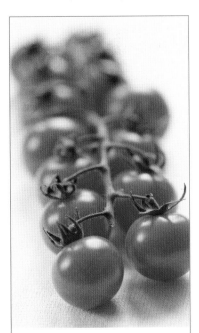

17 3 oz canned **tuna** in brine mixed with 1 teaspoon of low-fat mayonnaise and 1 scallion, chopped.

18 About 30 small black or green **olives** or 10 large chili-stuffed olives.

19 One slice of **fruit toast** (around 1 inch thick) spread with a little low-fat spread.

20 Six **cherry tomatoes** served with 2 cheese-spread triangles.

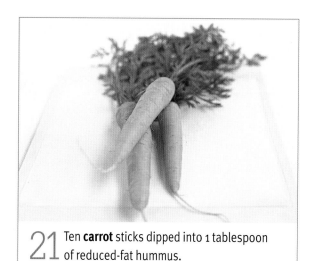

HEALTH BOOSTER

If you choose one of the juice- or smoothie-based recommendations as your morning snack (or start your breakfast or another meal with a freshly squeezed juice), don't wait too long before you drink it. Fresh juices start to lose their nutrients within ten minutes of being made, as the air starts to destroy the vital antioxidants within them.

21 Ten **carrot** sticks dipped into 1 tablespoon of reduced-fat hummus.

22 Half a **red bell pepper** dipped in 1 serving of Jerusalem Artichoke Hummus (see recipe on page 53).

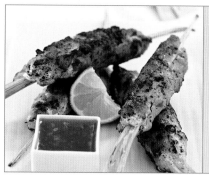

23 Two **Lemon Grass Fish Skewers** (see recipe on page 50) dipped into 1 teaspoon of sweet chili sauce or a low-fat yogurt based dip like tzatsiki.

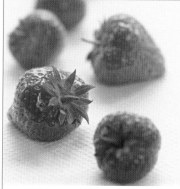

24 ¹/₄ cup low-fat **Greek or plain yogurt** sprinkled with 1 tablespoon of low-sugar granola.

25 **Roast beef roll-ups** — 3 slices of roast beef from the deli section of the supermarket wrapped around slices of red, yellow or green peppers.

26 Small carton of low-fat yogurt of any flavour served with 2 handfuls of **strawberries** or blueberries.

27 Three **crabsticks** served with 1 tablespoon of low-fat coleslaw.

28 Small carton of low-fat **plain yogurt** served with any piece of fruit.

29 Two **rye crackers** topped with 1 oz low-fat pâté.

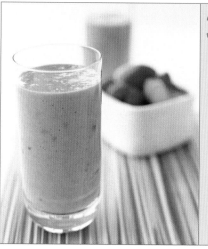

30 One **Fruity Summer Milkshake** (see recipe on page 52). You can replace the straw-berries and/or raspberries in this recipe with any other soft berry such as blueberries, blackcurrants, blackberries, or cherries.

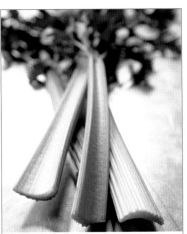

31 One mini gouda-type light **cheese** and 1 small fruit such as an apricot or plum.

32 1 oz low-fat **brie cheese** with 3 small pickled gherkins.

33 One **egg** boiled, then mashed and mixed with a little mustard. Serve with 2 celery sticks.

REMINDER

Don't forget to accompany each of your snacks with a glass of water, green tea, herbal tea, or low-calorie soda to keep your hydration levels up. One of the most common mistakes made by dieters is to mistake signals of thirst for hunger, so keep drinking those fluids regularly throughout the day.

34 Two **celery** sticks topped with 1 tablespoon of baba ganoush or low-fat hummus.

35 Two **Melba toasts** topped with 2 tablespoons ricotta cheese and 1 teaspoon of low-sugar jelly.

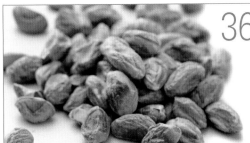

36 A very small handful of **pistachios,** peanuts, or cashews. Choose unsalted or un-roasted varieties where possible.

37 One **pancake** topped with 1 tablespoon of low-fat aerosol cream and a few berries.

38 Two flavored **rice cakes** served with $2/3$ cup skim or soy milk.

39 Five **almonds** and 3 dried apricots.

DO YOU NEED A FOOD DIARY?

The three snacks you eat each day on this plan will help reduce your risk of one of the biggest problems many dieters experience. It is called eating amnesia, and its symptoms are forgetting about snacks and treats you've nibbled throughout the day and then wondering why you're not getting the results you think you should be. When most dieters are asked what they ate in a day, they only remember around 88 percent of the calories they consume, and the calories they have forgotten total about 400 a day (more than enough to cut possible weight loss down from $2^1/4$ lb a week to just a few ounces).

Because you have regular snack times on this plan you are less likely to nibble between meals because you are already eating every 2–3 hours. However, if you aren't getting the results you expect or your weight loss starts to slow down after two or three weeks, try keeping a food diary recording everything that goes into your mouth as soon as you've eaten it. In this way you can spot any mindless calories you might be consuming: potential danger spots are foods nibbled while you clear away leftovers or bites taken while cooking.

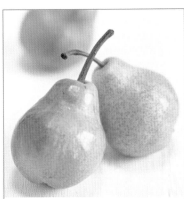

40 An apple or **pear** halved then spread with 1 teaspoon of peanut butter.

Mid-morning snack recipes

Try these tasty and nutritious options if you want something more exotic for your mid-morning break or want to make a batch of snacks to store in the refrigerator to take to work each day. None are complicated or time-consuming to prepare.

Smoked salmon thai rolls

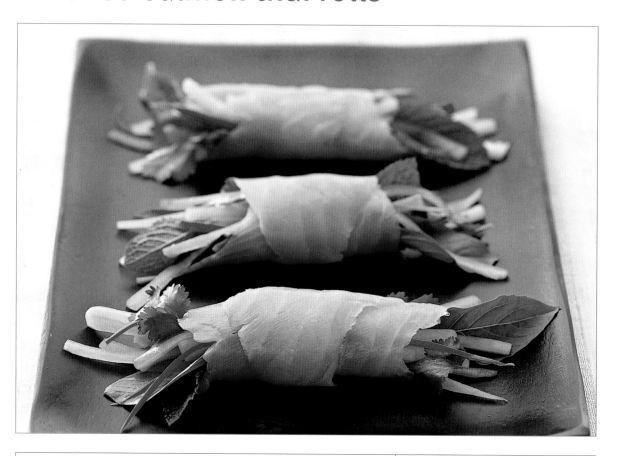

Makes 12
Preparation time 15 minutes

Nutritional values
Calories 32
Kilojoules 134
Protein 2 g
Carbohydrates 4 g
Fat 1 g

12 slices of smoked salmon

1 cucumber, peeled, seeded, and cut into matchsticks

1 long red chili, seeded, and thinly sliced

handful each of cilantro, mint, and Thai basil leaves

DRESSING

2 tablespoons sweet chili sauce

2 tablespoons honey

2 tablespoons lime juice

1 tablespoon nam pla (Thai fish sauce)

1 Separate the smoked salmon slices and lay them flat on a work surface. Arrange the cucumber, chili and herbs on the smoked salmon slices, placing an equal mound on each slice.

2 Combine the dressing ingredients and drizzle over the cucumber, chili and herb filling.

3 Roll up the salmon slices to enclose the filling and dressing and serve.

Good fats

Smoked salmon is one of the best sources of omega-3 fats which researchers in the Czech Republic have found actually decrease the number of fat cells we have in our bodies (and prevents those we do have from getting too large). If it's easier to make these rolls one or two at a time, do it by adding a few slices of cucumber and chili and a sprinkle of each herb and store any left-over dressing in an airtight jar in the refrigerator.

Diet power-up

If you work in an office where people regularly nip out to pick up snacks, it can be tricky to turn these down. Try these three tactics:

Make yourself a cheat jar Put some money in a jar on your desk every time you weaken and donate it to charity at the end of the month. Exactly how much you fine yourself is up to you — but the higher the fine, the more of a deterrent it will be.

Try a reward jar If you prefer positive reinforcement, put cash in your jar or stick a gold star on your computer that is worth a set monetary amount every time you say no to temptation. At the end of the month you can buy yourself a reward with the cash.

Schedule a bathroom break If the snack call at your office goes out at 11 a.m., make sure you're not at your desk. Or ask the order-taker to not stop by your desk for a while.

Bloody marianna

2 celery sticks, plus extra to serve (optional)

$^1/_4$ cucumber

12 oz tomatoes

$^1/_2$ red bell pepper, cored and seeded

1 apple

2–3 sprigs of mint

Worcestershire sauce, to taste

Tabasco sauce, to taste

crushed ice, to serve

1 Cut all the vegetables and fruit into chunks and feed them through a juicer or liquidizer and mix them with the mint.

2 Add the Worcestershire and Tabasco sauces to the mixture to taste and stir.

3 Pour the liquid into two glasses half-filled with ice and serve with celery-stick stirrers, if desired.

Do you eat five-plus a day?

Research from Pennsylvania State University indicates that one of the biggest predictors for successful weight loss was eating at least five portions of fruit and vegetables a day. Most people don't manage this, but if you ensure that at least one of your snacks each day contains one serving of fruit or vegetables (the Bloody Marianna on this page contains two if you eat the celery stirrers) this, combined with the high fruit and vegetable content of your main meals, will ensure that you manage your recommended dose. Remember, a portion of fruit or vegetables is:

• One large slice of fruit such as melon, pineapple, or mango
• One medium piece of fruit such as apple or orange
• Two pieces of a small fruit such as apricot or kiwifruit
• Two handfuls of berries
• One handful of dried fruit
• One glass of fruit or vegetable juice
• Two handfuls of any vegetable or bean.

Serves 2
Preparation time 5 minutes

Nutritional values
Calories 72
Kilojoules 302
Protein 2 g
Carbohydrates 13 g
Fat 1 g

Parmesan and herb scones

2 cups self-rising flour, plus extra for dusting

1/3 cup unsalted butter, diced

4 tablespoons grated Parmesan cheese

3 tablespoons chopped mixed fresh herbs
(such as oregano and chives)

1 egg, lightly beaten

2 tablespoons buttermilk

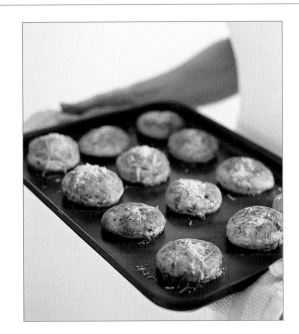

1 Sift the flour into a large bowl, add the butter, and blend with the fingertips until the mixture resembles fine bread crumbs. Add 3 tablespoons of the Parmesan and the herbs and stir together.

2 Beat together the egg and buttermilk. Use a knife or fork to combine the wet and dry ingredients lightly and bring them together to form a ball.

3 Shape the dough into a round, about 1 inch thick, and press out 12 rounds with a plain 2 inch cutter.

4 Place the rounds on a lightly floured baking sheet and sprinkle over the reserved Parmesan. Cook in a preheated oven, 425°F, for 10–12 minutes until golden and well risen. The scones can be stored in an airtight container for up to 3 days.

Makes 12
Preparation time 10 minutes
Cooking time 12 minutes

Nutritional values
Calories 128
Kilojoules 537
Protein 3 g
Carbohydrates 14 g
Fat 7 g

Lemon grass fish skewers

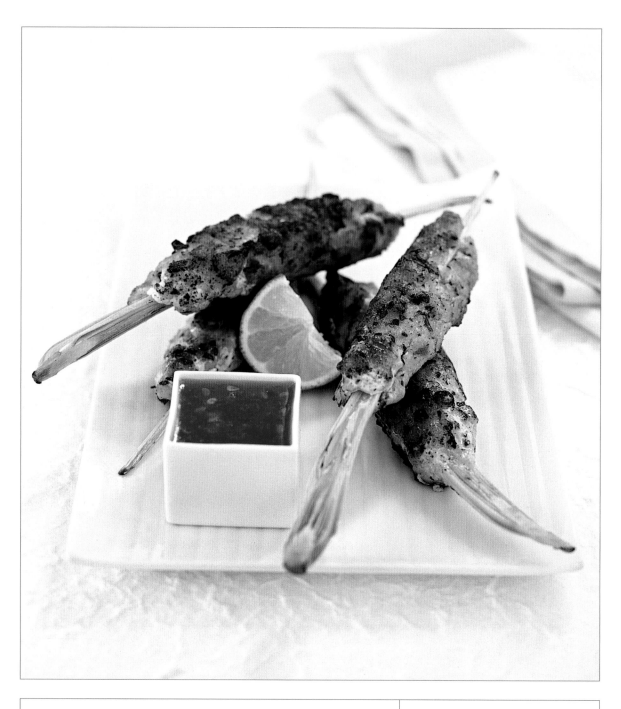

Makes 4
Preparation time 5 minutes
Cooking time 5 minutes

Nutritional values
Calories 55
Kilojoules 231
Protein 8 g
Carbohydrates 0 g
Fat 1 g

8 oz haddock, boned, skinned, and cut into small pieces

$^1/_2$ tablespoon mint

1 tablespoon cilantro

1 teaspoon Thai red curry paste

1 lime leaf, finely chopped, or the zest of 1 lime

2 lemon grass stalks, quartered lengthwise

oil, for brushing

sweet chili sauce, to serve

1 Place the fish, mint, cilantro, curry paste, and lime leaf or zest in a blender or food processor and blend for 15–30 seconds until well combined.

2 Divide the mixture into 8 and form each around a lemon grass stalk "skewer". Brush with a little oil, then place under a preheated hot grill and cook for 4–5 minutes until cooked through. Serve immediately.

Skewered snack

This recipe may seem far too complicated as a morning snack but a set of skewers will be okay refrigerated for 24 hours. You could have them as an evening meal choice, reserving two for your morning snack the next day. Try serving the skewers with $^1/_4$ cup couscous or rice and 2 tablespoons of salsa or guacamole on the side. Don't forget to increase the recipe quantity if you're cooking for more than just yourself.

Three simple tone-ups, no gym required

Aerobic exercise doesn't need to take place in the gym to impact on your weight loss. Next time you have a spare 60 seconds try one of these three simple exercises:

Tummy toner Sit upright in your chair, feet flat on the floor. Now slowly contract your tummy muscles so you are pulling your navel back towards your spine. Hold for 30–60 seconds then slowly release.

Bottom firmer While sitting at your desk or the dining table, clench and unclench your bottom muscles up to 50 times. Try this with your legs pressed tightly together to engage your inner and outer thigh muscles.

Calf toners While standing slowly raise yourself up and down on your tip toes. Try to ensure that your weight transfers over your big toes instead of the outside of your foot.

Fruity summer milkshake

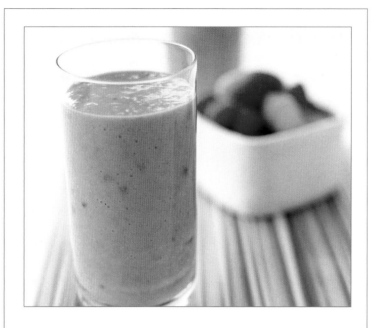

Smoothie tip

Research by Dr Barbara Rolls at Pennsylvania State University has found that the longer you whip up a smoothie and the more air that is incorporated into the blend the more filling that smoothie is going to be. If you're making up a blended snack like the Summer Milkshake here, beat the ingredients for at least one minute to create a fluffier, more filling treat. Also, avoid gulping down any purely liquid snacks as this will prevent them registering in the satiety part of your brain — sip them slowly or even drink half then take a short break to prolong the length of time you're "eating."

1 ripe peach, halved, pitted, and chopped

1 cup strawberries

1^1/$_4$ cups raspberries

1 cup soy milk

ice cubes, to serve

1 Put the peach in a blender or food processor with the strawberries and raspberries and blend to a smooth purée, scraping the mixture down from the sides of the bowl if necessary.

2 Add the soy milk and blend the ingredients again until the mixture is smooth and frothy. Pour the milkshake over the ice cubes in tall glasses.

Serves 2
Preparation time 2 minutes

Nutritional values
Calories 90
Kilojoules 380
Protein 5 g
Carbohydrates 2 g
Fat 2 g

Jerusalem artichoke hummus

12 oz Jerusalem artichokes, scrubbed

$^1/_4$ cup butter, diced

$^2/_3$ cup chicken stock

8 oz canned chickpeas, drained

1 teaspoon ground cumin

2 tablespoons lemon juice

1 garlic clove, crushed

1 Place the artichokes in a pan of boiling water and cook for 5 minutes or until tender. Drain and let cool.

2 Put the artichokes in a blender or food processor with the butter and stock and process until smooth. Add the chickpeas, cumin, lemon juice, and garlic and process again until smooth.

Beware transition time

Have you ever noticed that some tense moments you have with family members or work colleagues occur first thing in the morning as you rush to go to work or as soon as you walk in the door at night? If you do you're not alone: these points, known as transition times, have been identified by stress experts as major flare points throughout the day. Why are you being told this within a diet book? Because anger is a major comfort-eating trigger, actually ranking above stress for women who often find it a tricky emotion to let out.

Dr Redford Williams from Duke University Medical Center in Durham, North Carolina, has found people who score highest in measures of anger also score highest in energy consumption, eating 600 more calories (2520 kj) a day than calmer types. To try and ease your transition to work each morning and back home at night, spend 2–3 minutes of your journey thinking about nothing except what you can see, hear or smell around you. This helps you create a break from home and work and makes the switch from either environment easier to handle.

Serves 6
Preparation time 10 minutes
Cooking time 5 minutes

Nutritional values
Calories 69
Kilojoules 290
Carbohydrates 12 g
Fat 1 g
Protein 4 g

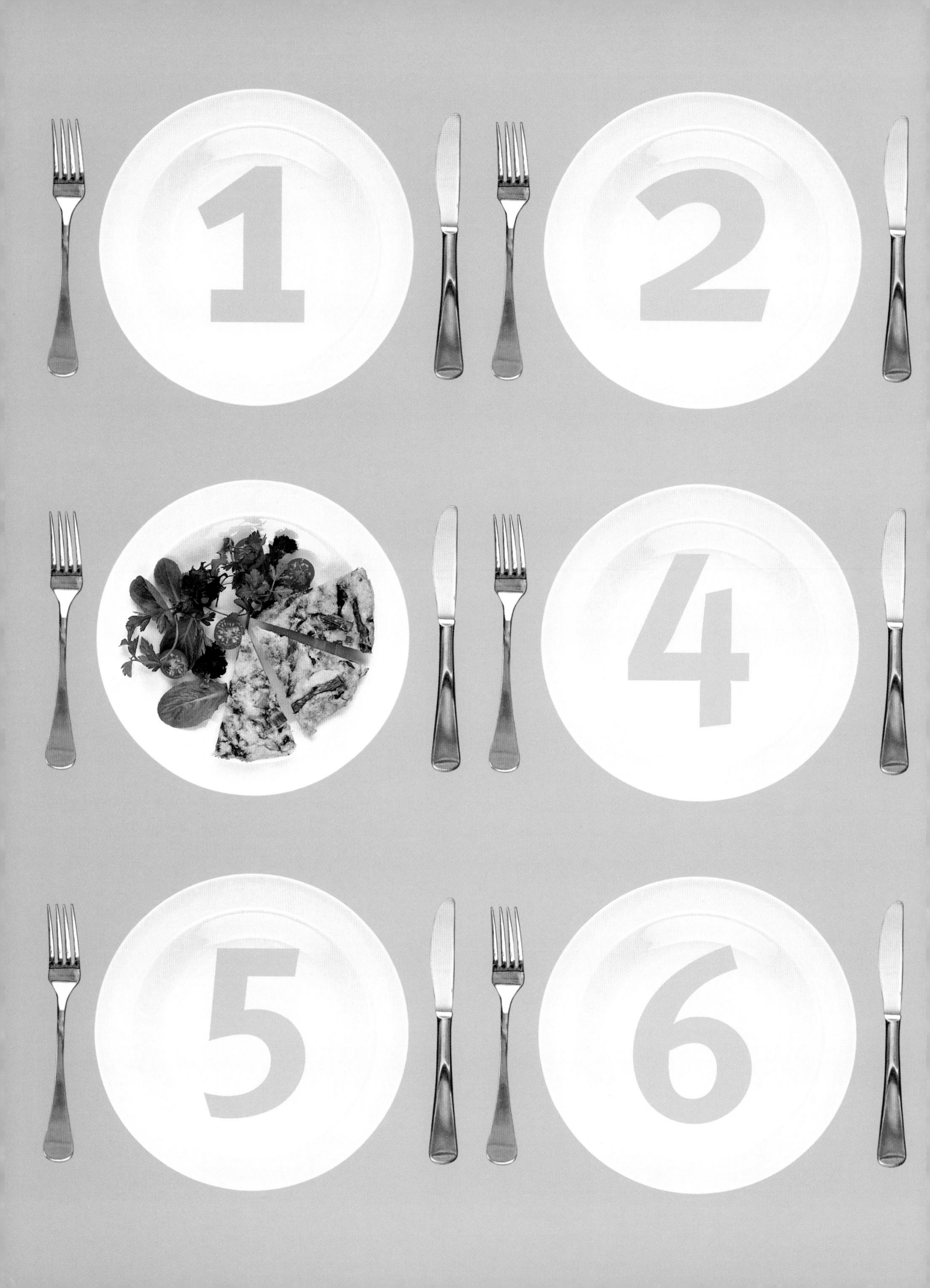
1
2
4
5
6

Lunch

There was a time when lunch was an important meal — work would stop, people would sit down at a real table and eat a healthy meal that would sustain them for the rest of the day. This is no longer the case.

According to the American Dietetic Association, two-thirds of US workers eat lunch at their desk at least once a week, while other studies have found that the average American skips lunch 59 times a year. In the UK the average "lunch hour" lasts just 36 minutes. The fact is, many of us now see lunch as something that should be got out of the way so we can continue with the rest of our day.

But this lunch-is-for-wimps ethos is potentially one of the main causes of our weight-gain battles. If you skip lunch or eat a meal high in refined carbohydrates (like the white bread sandwich and bag of potato chips many of us consume) your body will be subject to the same blood-sugar seesaw discussed in the breakfast section. Combine this with the fact that after lunch your body's energy naturally takes a dip and it's clear to see why so many of us start reaching for sugary snacks at 3 p.m. But the solution isn't to indulge in a huge lunch either. If you eat too heavy a meal, blood that should be taking energizing oxygen to your brain is diverted to your stomach and you end up feeling sleepy, sluggish and again, reaching for sugary or caffeinated treats to re-energize yourself. Getting the balance right at lunchtime is therefore important, not only to fuel your working day, but also to keep you on track for your weight loss.

So what is the perfect balance? As with breakfast, you need a good mix of protein and carbohydrates, firstly to balance your energy levels, but also to provide your brain with the perfect mix of calming serotonin (produced when we eat carbohydrates) and stimulating dopamine (from proteins) that helps promote concentration, motivation, and problem-solving skills. As for the size of the meal, most nutritional experts say that the perfect lunch contains between 400–750 calories (anything over 800 calories is likely to tax your digestion enough to cause fatigue) and is low in saturated fats that the body finds hard to digest.

Choose from 50 lunches

Each lunch is around 450 calories which is hefty enough to satisfy your appetite, but light enough to avoid overloading your digestion leading to afternoon fatigue (and the sugar cravings that come with it). There are a variety of meal types, so that there is a choice for any kind of day: whether you're at home, in an office with a refrigerator and microwave, or have to rely on a lunchbox, canteen, or fast food restaurant.

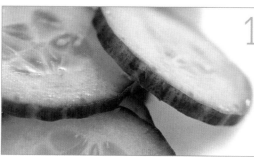

1 A **salad** of unlimited sliced cucumber, tomato, and red onion topped with 10 olives and 2 oz low-fat feta cheese.

2 One medium **vegetable samosa** around 6 oz. Served with a side salad of grated carrot and 1 teaspoon of raisins topped with 1 tablespoon of tzatsiki.

3 **Omelet** made from 2 eggs and filled with your choice of sliced red bell pepper, mushrooms, tomatoes, onion, or zucchini. Serve with 2 pieces of multigrain toast.

4 4 oz broiled **chicken breast** or 3 tablespoons of low-fat hummus served with Tabbouleh (either made from the recipe on page 64 or an 8 oz serving from the supermarket deli counter).

5 4 oz **roast chicken, pork, or lean beef** served with unlimited cauliflower, cabbage, and carrots plus 2 small roasted potatoes or 4 oz potatoes mashed with a little low-fat milk. Top with 1 tablespoon of gravy.

ARE YOU A DESK POTATO?

The term used to describe people who get to work, sit down, and don't actually leave their desk (except for bathroom breaks) until the end of the day — and just like the couch potato, the result is weight gain. Try to get outside and take a lunchtime walk for at least 10–15 minutes each day if you can. You will burn 50–100 calories, and according to weight-loss experts, that's enough to prevent the 5–10 lb the average person puts on each decade and blames on their age.

6 One **hot dog** roll filled with 1 frankfurter or vegetarian sausage and half an onion fried using an oil spray. Add mustard and ketchup to taste. Serve with a small bag of low-fat potato chips.

7 Ready-meal **lasagna** (meat or vegetarian) or other pasta dish under 350 calories served with an Italian salad of sliced tomatoes, some fresh basil, and a drizzle of 1 teaspoon of olive oil.

8 8 oz **baked potato** (roughly the size of a computer mouse), topped with 3 tablespoons of baked beans and 3 tablespoons grated cheese or 3 tablespoons of low-fat coleslaw.

**WHY LEISURELY LUNCHES
MAKE YOU THIN**
Taking your time over lunch and chewing everything well will help your weight loss further. When you chew, the mouth sends messages to the brain about what type of food it has eaten and how much. When your brain believes it has had enough, it sends fullness signals to your stomach. If you don't chew correctly, these signals aren't as strong and you eat more than you need.

9 Small **multigrain roll** filled with 2 oz canned tuna in brine or salmon and slices of cucumber. Serve with 2 handfuls of baby carrots dipped in 2 tablespoons of salsa.

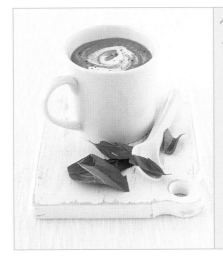

10 Bowl of **Roasted Red Pepper and Tomato Soup** (see recipe on page 62). Serve with a small wholewheat pita bread dipped in 3 tablespoons of reduced-fat hummus.

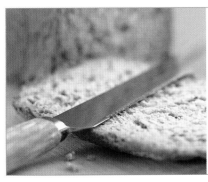

11 Two slices of **multigrain bread** topped with 2 slices of lean ham or half a red bell pepper (broiled if possible) and 1 oz brie. Add some arugula leaves and serve with 3–4 celery sticks.

12 Six pieces of **sushi**, any fillings, served with a cup of miso soup. You'll find sachets of this in Asian stores and some large supermarkets.

13 **Coleslaw-style salad** made from unlimited grated cabbage, cauliflower, and onion mixed with 1 tablespoon low-fat mayonnaise. Top with 3 slices of lean roast beef or 3 tablespoons grated cheese.

14 One serving of **Thai Tofu Cakes** (see recipe on page 65) served with a salad made from raw broccoli, red bell pepper and baby corn. Serve with 2 teaspoons of sweet chili sauce.

15 Two **Melba toasts** spread with 2 tablespoons cream cheese and topped with 2 oz smoked salmon. Serve with half an avocado, sliced.

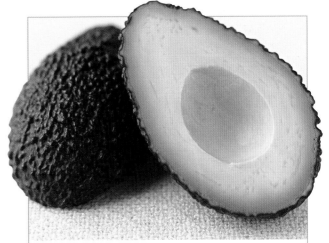

16 Half an **avocado** topped with 6 crabsticks, mixed with 1 tablespoon of low-calorie salad dressing. Serve with slices of red, yellow, and green bell peppers.

THE EASIEST WAY TO INCREASE NUTRIENT INTAKE

Many of us choose our lunch by whatever is quick, easy, and available, but to truly boost your health you should choose something you really enjoy. Why? Researchers in the 1970s gave a group of Swedish women and a group of Thai women a spicy curry to eat; the Thai women, who enjoyed the dish, absorbed up to 50 percent more iron from the dish than the Swedish women who found it too hot for their taste. It seems that the anticipation of a meal or snack triggers the production of digestive juices slightly earlier in the eating process which ensures that food is well broken down when it reaches the intestines where nutrients are absorbed. Whatever you choose to eat on this plan make it something you really enjoy, and spend a few minutes before you eat thinking about what you are consuming.

17 One **Lebanese flatbread** spread with 1 tablespoon of tzatziki and filled with grated carrot, onion, and sliced beet. Serve with 2 tablespoons of chickpeas mixed with a little cilantro.

18 Two slices of **multigrain or rye toast** topped with 7 oz baked beans.

19 **Salad** of unlimited celery and apple chopped into small pieces and mixed with 1 tablespoon of raisins and 2 tablespoons of chopped walnuts. Add $^1/_2$ oz crumbled Stilton and mix well.

20 **Triple-decker club** sandwich made from 3 slices of bread spread with a little mustard. Fill with 2 slices of lean ham, 2 slices of chicken breast, 2 slices of processed cheese, and 1 tomato, sliced. Serve with 6 pickled onions and a handful of carrot sticks.

21 Four **stuffed vine leaves** (from the supermarket deli counter) served with $^1/_3$ cup couscous made to package instructions and cooled. Serve with 1 tablespoon of baba ganoush or low-fat hummus.

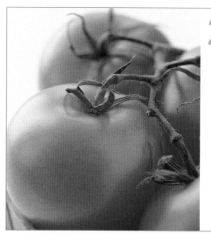

22 **Tomato and mozzarella salad** made from 2–3 sliced tomatoes and 2 oz low-fat buffalo mozzarella. Add 1 teaspoon of pesto sauce to the side and serve with 2 Melba toasts.

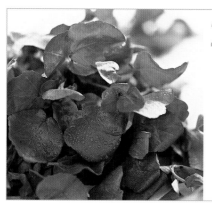

23 **Summer salad** made from unlimited watercress and orange and beetroot slices. Top with 3 slices of parma ham or 2 handfuls of sunflower seeds.

24 One **bagel** halved, top each half with a quarter of an avocado, mashed, half a tomato, sliced, and 1 well-broiled Canadian bacon slice or 2 vegetarian slices.

25 Any 350-calorie or under **ready-made sandwich** served with a small bag of low-fat chips.

26 One serving of **French Bread Pizza with Salami** (see recipe on page 69) served with a salad of arugula with balsamic vinegar.

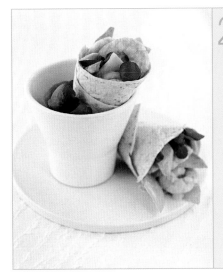

27 Two slices of **toast** topped with 1 can (around 4 oz) of sardines in tomato sauce. Serve with a salad of watercress and cucumber.

28 One serving of **Shrimp, Mango, and Avocado Wrap** (see recipe on page 66) served with a salad of arugula or baby spinach leaves and sliced red bell pepper topped with a little balsamic vinegar or other low-fat dressing.

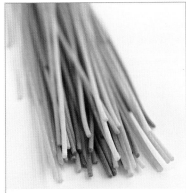

29 4 oz slice of any **quiche** served with 5 oz baked beans or unlimited amounts of any green vegetable.

30 Any **ready meal** under 350 calories served with a side salad of tomato and onion topped with 1 tablespoon of low-calorie salad dressing.

31 50 g (2 oz) **spaghetti** cooked as per instructions then tossed with 25 g (1 oz) grated cheese, 8 chopped olives and 1 tablespoon of olive oil.

32 Four **oatcakes** served with 2oz pâté and 1 oz low-fat cheese. Add 2 tablespoons of relish and 1 handful of baby carrots.

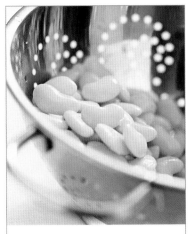

33 One serving of **Pasta Salad with Crab, Lemon, and Arugula** (see recipe on page 68). Serve with 1 slice of toasted multigrain bread or 2 oatcakes.

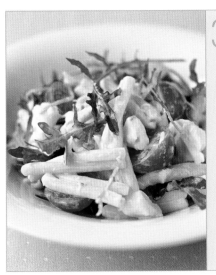

34 $1/4$ cup **lima beans** or kidney beans added to any 10 oz can of vegetable soup before heating. Serve with 2 slices of multigrain bread.

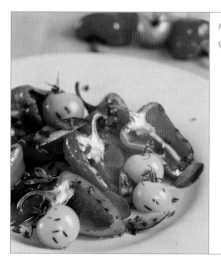

35 One panini bread filled with a selection of **roasted vegetables**, or topped with 3 oz antipasti from the supermarket deli counter. Drain this well as it can be oily.

36 One **tortilla wrap** spread with salsa and topped with 3 tablespoons grated cheese, 2 tablespoons cooked, canned kidney beans, and 1 slice of turkey breast or 2 slices of vegetarian ham. Fold into a burrito and eat cold or microwave for 45 seconds to melt the cheese.

37 One medium (around 3 oz) **sausage roll**, either meat or vegetarian served with 3 tablespoons of low-fat coleslaw.

38 One small fast-food **hamburger or cheeseburger** served with a salad (choose the no- or low-calorie dressing option).

39 4 oz **new potatoes** chopped and mixed with 2 scallions, chopped, 2 Canadian or vegetarian bacon slices, well broiled and 1 egg, boiled and sliced. Add 1 tablespoon of low-fat mayonnaise.

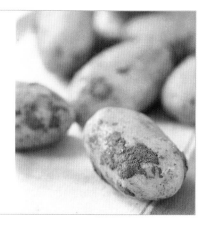

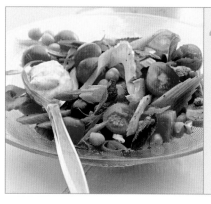

40 One serving of **Chickpea and Olive Salad** (see recipe on page 72) served with half a bagel spread with a little hummus.

41 One small **pita bread** spread with 2 tablespoons low-fat cream cheese and filled with 3 sun-dried tomatoes, chopped. Serve with a cup of Roasted Red Pepper and Tomato Soup (see page 62) or 10 oz can of tomato or vegetable soup.

42 **Shrimp cocktail** made from 3 oz fresh shrimp mixed with 1 tablespoon of low-calorie dressing and diced cucumber. Serve with 2 slices of multigrain bread.

43 One serving of **Baked Vegetable Frittata** (see recipe on page 73) served with a green salad.

44 One **English muffin** topped with 1 egg, poached and 1 tablespoon of hollandaise sauce. Serve with a salad of baby spinach.

THE FAT-BURNING SALAD DRESSING

Many of the lunch suggestions here are accompanied by salad. While any low-calorie salad dressing can be used, you can power up your weight loss by making a dressing with flaxseed oil, which contains essential fats that trigger fat burning. Mix 2 tablespoons of flaxseed oil, 2 tablespoons of lemon juice, and 3 tablespoons of balsamic vinegar in a jar and keep the jar in the refrigerator. Use 1 tablespoon at a time on salads or vegetables.

45 5 oz pot of low-fat **hummus** or 4 oz baba ganoush served with unlimited crudités of carrot, celery, and green bell pepper and 2 small wholewheat pita cut into slices.

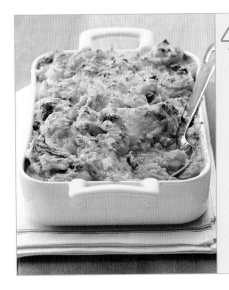

46 One serving of **Cheesy Lentil and Vegetable Pie** (see recipe on page 70) served with a small salad of lettuce leaves and thinly sliced cucumber.

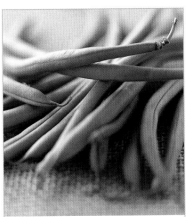

47 Five **falafel balls** served with 1 tablespoon of baba ganoush or salsa. Accompany with slices of cucumber, carrot, and yellow bell pepper.

48 Four **rye crackers** spread with $^1/_4$ cup low-fat cream cheese and top each with 1 slice of smoked salmon and serve with 2 small dill pickles.

49 **Niçoise-style salad** made from unlimited green beans and sliced tomato. Topped with 1 boiled egg, sliced, 2 oz canned tuna in brine and 6 black olives.

50 Three large **chicken satay** sticks (from the supermarket) dipped in 1 teaspoon of peanut butter. Serve with unlimited lettuce and celery.

THREE WAYS TO MAKE TIME FOR LUNCH

If you are guilty of skipping lunch because you don't think you have time to eat, think again. Freeing up even 30 minutes of your day to eat lunch will actually make you more accurate and productive in the afternoon.

Tidy your desk You waste an average of 7.5 hours a week looking for things you can't find on a messy desk. When sorting through things, use the three Ds — either Deal with a piece of paper (which might mean filing it, returning a call or putting it in an in tray to truly tackle later), Delegate it, or Dump it.

Learn to say no If you are too busy for lunch, you are too busy to take on someone else's work.

Make a to-do list People who make lists complete things a fifth faster; but a bad to-do list adds pressure. Stress experts say a list should have no more than four things on it at any one time, and these should be only those things that absolutely must be done today. Once you've completed those you can start adding additional tasks.

Lunch recipes

We sometimes get stuck in a lunchtime food rut, alternating between the same two or three meals each day. This is not only boring, it also reduces the diversity of nutrients we consume. On this plan try to eat a different thing for lunch each day and try some of these recipes, all of which can be prepared the night before and taken into the office in airtight containers.

Roasted red pepper and tomato soup

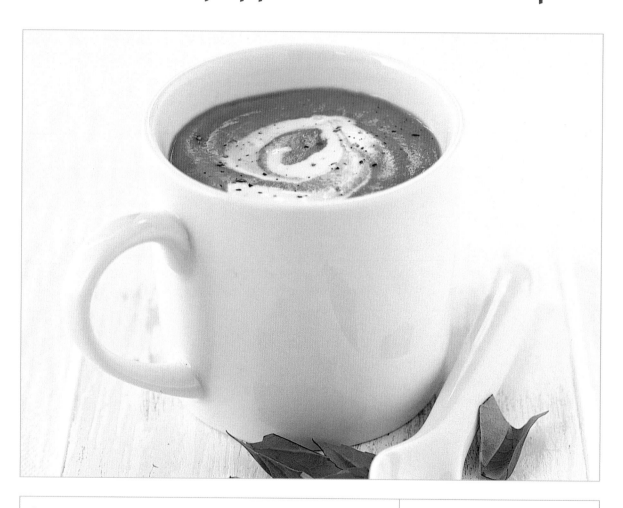

Serves 4
Preparation time 10 minutes
Cooking time 40 minutes

Nutritional values
Calories 96
Kilojoules 403
Protein 3 g
Carbohydrates 16 g
Fat 3 g

4 red bell peppers, cored and seeded

1 lb tomatoes, halved

1 teaspoon olive oil

1 onion, chopped

1 carrot, chopped

$2^1/_2$ cups vegetable stock

2 tablespoons sour cream

handful of basil, torn

salt and pepper

1 Place the peppers, skin side up, and the tomatoes, skin side down, on a baking sheet under a preheated hot broiler and cook for 8–10 minutes until the skins are blackened. Remove the peppers and place them in a plastic bag. Seal and let cool, then remove the skins and slice the flesh. Leave the tomatoes to cool and remove the skins.

2 Meanwhile, heat the oil in a large saucepan, add the onion and carrot and fry for 5 minutes. Add the vegetable stock, peppers, and tomatoes, bring to a boil and simmer for 25 minutes.

3 Transfer the mixture to a food processor or blender and blend until smooth. Stir through the sour cream and basil and season well. If you're making this for a weekend lunch, or work from home, serve immediately.

4 If you're taking this soup to work put it in a thermos flask to keep it warm, or put it in a microwavable container and warm it for 2 minutes before serving.

Antioxidants

The red colour of this soup indicates that it is an important source of a vital antioxidant nutrient called lycopene. Found in tomatoes, red bell peppers, watermelon, pink grapefruit, and other fruits with reddish hues, this has been linked to a lowered risk of heart disease and many cancers. Lycopene is absorbed better from cooked versions of the foods that contain it and you do need a little fat in the meal to help you absorb it, so don't be tempted to leave the olive oil or sour cream out of this recipe.

Eating out at lunchtime

If you have to eat out on this plan, you can still stick to your diet if you make the right choices.

Appetizers Skip them if you can, but if it would seem rude the three best choices are melon and prosciutto; any non-creamy soup (like gazpacho), or a simple seafood-based dish such as seared tuna or smoked salmon.

Main courses Best choices are lean proteins such as steak, fish, or chicken without sauces and served with plain vegetables or salad (dressing on the side). Pasta dishes with tomato or seafood sauces are also healthy, but watch the portion sizes.

Desserts Again, skip them if you can, but if not, good choices are fresh fruit, sorbets, or a small serving of crème caramel.

Tabbouleh

1¹/₃ cups bulgar wheat

4 scallions, finely chopped

4 tablespoons chopped mint

4 tablespoons chopped parsley

1 garlic clove, crushed

3 tablespoons olive oil

4 tablespoons lemon juice

10 oz cherry tomatoes, halved

pepper

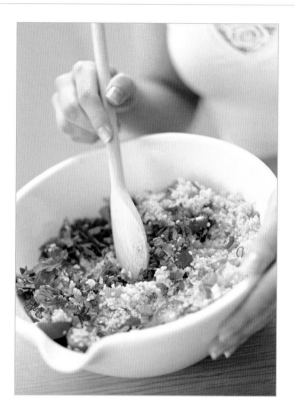

1 Place the bulgar wheat in a large heatproof bowl, cover with plenty of boiled water and let stand for 30 minutes. Drain well.

2 Stir in the scalloins, herbs, garlic, olive oil, lemon juice, and tomatoes. Season to taste.

3 If you're taking this to work, put it into an airtight container and refrigerate. Take the dish out 5–10 minutes before you want to eat it as it's best served at room temperature.

Serves 4
Preparation time 5 minutes, plus standing

Nutritional values
Calories 290
Kilojoules 1218
Protein 4 g
Carbohydrates 41 g
Fat 12 g

Thai tofu cakes

1 bunch of scallions, roughly chopped

1 inch piece of fresh ginger root, roughly chopped

1 lemon grass stalk, roughly chopped

4 garlic cloves

2 teaspoons superfine sugar

2 teaspoons nam pla (Thai fish sauce)

8 oz tofu

2 cups bread crumbs

1 egg white

3 tablespoons groundnut or soy bean oil

1 Put the scallions, ginger, lemon grass, garlic, sugar, and nam pla into a food processor. Blend the ingredients to a paste.

2 Break the tofu into pieces and add them to the paste together with the bread crumbs. Blend the mixture until just combined, add the egg white and blend again.

3 Shape dessertspoonfuls of the mixture into 4 flat cakes, lightly dusting your hands with a little flour if the mixture feels sticky.

4 Brush the cakes with a little oil and cook them in a large, heavy skillet, for about 2 minutes or until golden-brown. Turn them over and cook for an additional 1–2 minutes.

5 If you're taking this to work, refrigerate the cakes when all are cooked, then warm them in a microwave for 2 minutes or in a preheated oven, 400°F, for 10–15 minutes.

Strange but true

Some 26 percent of women and 10 percent of men spend their lunch breaks shopping, according to a study by British bread company Nimble. But if you are among them you may spend more than you think while on this eating plan. According to German scientists, women, in particular, like their bodies far more when they eat regularly. And this in turn helps your diet success — women who don't judge their bodies when they see them are 40 percent more likely to succeed on a diet plan than those who do pick out things they don't like. If you still find your eyes drawn to your hips or tummy when you look in the mirror, the Bach Flower remedy Crab Apple helps redress negative internal feelings.

Eating at your desk?

Eating at your desk is fine, but don't work or surf the Internet at the same time. Research reveals that people eat 15 percent more calories if they eat while distracted.

Serves 4
Preparation time 20 minutes
Cooking time 3-4 minutes

Nutritional values
Calories 295
Kilojoules 1240
Protein 6 g
Carbohydrates 25 g
Fat 12 g

Shrimp, mango, and avocado wrap

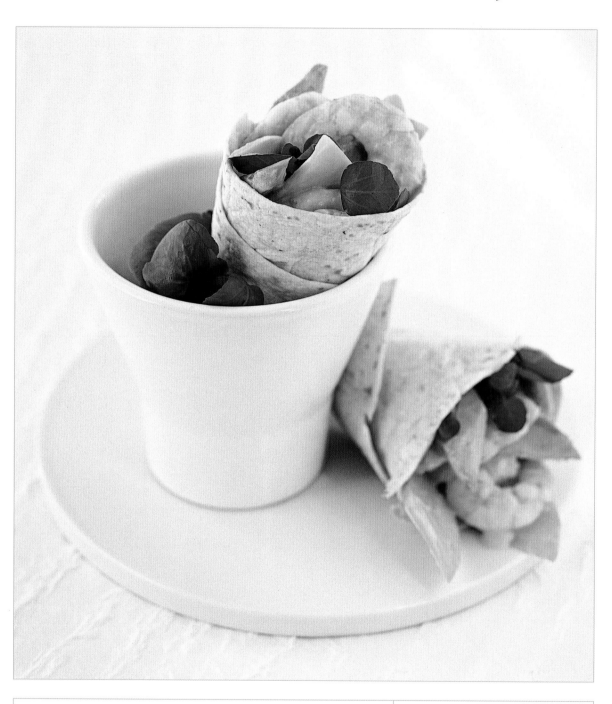

Serves 4
Preparation time 10 minutes

Nutritional values
Calories 314
Kilojoules 1318
Protein 19 g
Carbohydrates 32 g
Fat 12 g

2 tablespoons sour cream

2 teaspoons tomato ketchup

few drops of Tabasco sauce

10 oz cooked peeled shrimp

1 mango, peeled and thinly sliced

1 avocado, peeled and sliced

4 oz watercress

4 flour tortillas

1 In a medium bowl mix together the sour cream and ketchup. Add a few drops of Tabasco sauce to taste.

2 Add the shrimp, mango, and avocado and toss the mixture together. Divide the mixture among the tortillas, add some watercress, roll them up and serve.

3 If you're taking this recipe to work, don't make up the wrap until you get to the office or it will be too soggy to eat. Instead, put the shrimp mix in an airtight container and construct the tortilla at your desk or in the staff kitchen.

High GI?

Mangos have earned a bad reputation with dieters recently as they are a high GI fruit. However, when eaten with any form of protein or fat (as you do in this recipe) the speed at which they are turned to sugar in the body is slowed. This is good news as mangos are not only one of the tastiest fruits, they are also incredibly high in vitamin C, the antioxidant beta carotene, and potassium, a mineral we need for healthy hearts.

Is bread the best lunch option for you?

Many dieters cut bread out of their diet. However it is not bread itself that causes problems, but the type they are eating. White bread has a very high glycemic index and so creates high levels of blood sugar which then get shuttled into fat stores. Studies from Tufts University in the US have found that people eating white bread suffered a three times greater increase in their waist size each year than those eating wholegrains.

If, however, you suffer from bloating, fatigue, headaches or find that your weight increases by more than 2–3 lb the day after eating meals high in bread, it could be wheat causing problems. Try switching to wheat-free varieties of bread or pasta for a week or two. Most of the recipes here can be made with wheat-free products such as rye or gluten-free breads, cornstarch-based chapattis and oatcakes or rye crackers.

Pasta salad with crab, lemon, and arugula

2 oz dried pasta (such as rigatoni)

grated zest and juice of $^1/_2$ a lime

2 tablespoons plain yogurt

$3^1/_4$ oz canned crab meat, drained

8 cherry tomatoes, halved

handful of arugula leaves

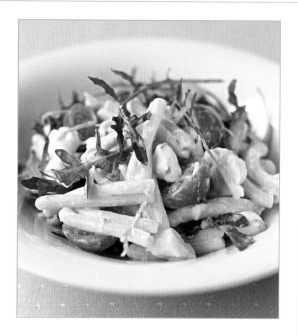

1 Cook the pasta according to the instructions on the packet and allow to cool.

2 In a large bowl mix together the lime zest and juice, yogurt and crab meat. Add the pasta and mix again.

3 Add the tomatoes and arugula to the bowl, toss everything together and serve.

4 If you're making this before work, stop after step 2, pack the arugula and tomato separately and add them just before you're ready to eat.

Serves 1
Preparation time 5 minutes, plus cooling
Cooking time 10 minutes

Nutritional values
Calories 330
Kilojoules 1386
Protein 22 g
Carbohydrates 49 g
Fat 6 g

French bread pizza with salami

1 baguette

6 tablespoons bottled tomato and basil pasta sauce

5 oz mozzarella cheese, sliced

3 oz pepperoni or salami, sliced

16 green olives, pitted and halved

1 teaspoon dried oregano

1 Cut the bread in half and split each piece horizontally to make 4 pieces. Place the bread, cut side up, on a baking sheet and spread the tomato and basil sauce over it.

2 Top with the mozzarella, pepperoni or salami, and olives and sprinkle with oregano.

3 Cook in a preheated oven, 400°F, for 5–6 minutes until the cheese has melted.

4 If you're taking this to work, wrap it in foil after cooking and either eat cold or reheat in the microwave.

Quick question

I really can't take any kind of food to work with me and have to rely on either the work canteen or local sandwich bar to make my lunch. Can I still stick to the plan?

Any sandwich bar or canteen can provide you with diet food if you know what to look for. Good choices are sandwiches that are made with unbuttered breads and mayonnaise-free tuna in brine, shrimp, chicken, ham, or roast beef with lots of salad or a little pickle. Or choose baked potatoes topped with around 3 tablespoons of baked beans, cottage cheese, vegetable chili, or ratatouille. Remember though, a healthy potato portion is about the size of a computer mouse; if your canteen only sells superssize, cut half off and throw it away before you start eating (a tactic that's much easier to do than leaving some on your plate). The same approach can be used if they add spoonful after spoonful of baked beans, just throw some away or push them to the side of your plate and cover them with salt so you can't eat them.

Serves 4
Preparation time 5 minutes
Cooking time 6 minutes

Nutritional values
Calories 324
Kilojoules 1360
Protein 18 g
Carbohydrates 38 g
Fat 11g

Cheesy lentil and vegetable pie

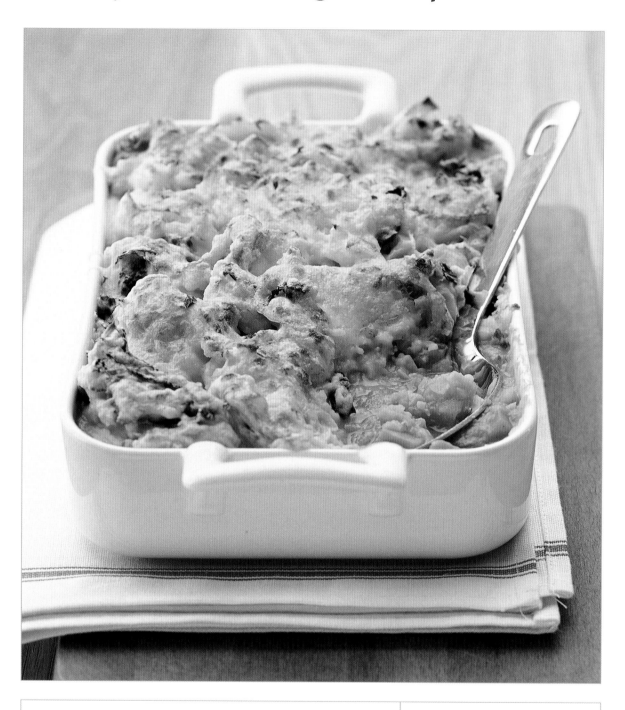

Serves 4
Preparation time 30 minutes
Cooking time 35 minutes

Nutritional values
Calories 480
Kilojoules 2016
Protein 25 g
Carbohydrates 68 g
Fat 14 g

1 tablespoon sunflower oil

1 onion, finely chopped

1 lb carrots, diced

2 garlic cloves, finely chopped

13$^1/_2$ oz can low-sugar, low-salt baked beans

$^1/_2$ cup red lentils

2 cups vegetable stock

salt and pepper

TOPPING

1$^1/_2$ lb baking potatoes

1$^1/_4$ cups finely shredded savoy cabbage

3–4 tablespoons low-fat milk

1 cup grated cheddar cheese

1 Heat the oil in a saucepan, add the onion and cook, stirring occasionally, for about 5 minutes or until softened.

2 Stir in the carrots and garlic and cook for 2 minutes. Mix in the baked beans, lentils, and stock and season to taste. Bring to a boil, cover, and simmer for 20 minutes until the lentils are tender, adding extra liquid if necessary.

3 Meanwhile, make the topping. Cut the potatoes into large chunks and cook them in the base of a steamer, half-filled with boiling water, for 15 minutes. Add the steamer top, fill with the cabbage, cover, and cook for 5 minutes until both cabbage and potatoes are tender.

4 Drain the potatoes, return them to the pan and mash with the milk. Stir in the cabbage and two-thirds of the cheese.

5 Spoon the hot carrot mixture into the base of a 6 cup pie dish. Spoon the potato mixture on top then sprinkle with the remaining cheese. Place under a preheated hot broiler for 5 minutes until golden-brown.

Packed with goodness

This dish is incredibly high in vitamins and minerals, not just because it is packed with vegetables and legumes, but also because it retains a high level of nutrients during cooking. Traditionally, when you boil vegetables, many of the nutrients within them leach into the cooking water. In this recipe the water (and the nutrients) are absorbed by the lentils. Other vegetables are also cooked in a steamer, which retains more nutrients than boiling. If you don't have a steamer boil the potatoes and cabbage in as little water as possible and only add them when the water is piping hot.

Starving even after your snack

You might be more sensitive than most people to the drop in hunger hormones cholecystokinin and glucagon that occurs in each of us shortly before midday. If you find you are ravenous at lunch and that the serving sizes here aren't enough for you, then either choose one of the nut-based mid-morning snacks or add 1 teaspoon of peanut butter to whatever snack you do choose (it will add some calories but probably less than you will consume by eating to excess at lunchtime). Researchers at the University of California have found that nut products seem to balance the hormone levels more effectively than any other food.

Chickpea and olive salad

1 lb 10 oz canned cooked chickpeas, drained

7 oz cherry tomatoes, halved

4 celery sticks, sliced

$^1/_3$ cup Kalamata olives, whole, rinsed well
   and drained

4 scallions, finely chopped

2 tablespoons tzatziki

pepper

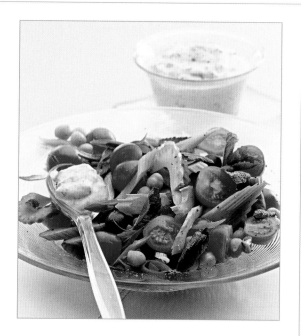

1 Put the chickpeas, cherry tomatoes, celery,
olives, and scallions in a serving bowl and
mix well.

2 Stir in the tzatziki, season with pepper to taste
and serve.

3 If you're taking this dish to work stop at the end
of step 1 and add the dressing only 1–2 minutes
before you intend to eat.

Serves 4
Preparation time 15 minutes

Nutritional values
Calories 248
Kilojoules 1041
Protein 19 g
Carbohydrates 19 g
Fat 4 g

Baked vegetable frittata

8 oz asparagus, trimmed and halved

1 tablespoon extra virgin olive oil

2 leeks, trimmed and sliced

2 garlic cloves, crushed

2 tablespoons chopped basil

6 eggs

2 tablespoons milk

2 tablespoons grated Parmesan cheese

salt and pepper

1 Cook the asparagus in a saucepan of lightly salted boiling water for 2 minutes, drain and shake dry.

2 Meanwhile, heat the oil in a large skillet and gently fry the leeks and garlic for 5 minutes or until they have softened. Add the asparagus and basil and remove the pan from the heat.

3 Beat the eggs with the milk and season with salt and pepper. Stir in the vegetable mixture and pour into a greased 5 cup ovenproof dish.

4 Scatter over the Parmesan and cook in a preheated oven, 400°F, for 15–20 minutes until firm in the center. Serve immediately.

Time for lunch?

Do you always have lunch at the same time each day? If you can manage this for other meals and snacks too, you could power up your weight loss. Recent research from Dr Hamid Farschi at the University of Nottingham in the UK, has discovered that women who eat at the same time each day actually burn up the calories they consume more rapidly then women who eat at irregular times.

Don't be afraid to bring your lunch

If you work in an office you may feel self-conscious about bringing in lunch. Rest easy. Studies by the American Restaurant Association found that 50 percent of workers take lunch to work each day with everything from sandwiches to last night's leftovers on the menu. Try packing moist items (salad dressings, spreads such as hummus, or wet vegetables such as tomatoes) separately and add them to meals at the last minute, and keep a plate or salad bowl in your office drawer so that you can eat using proper crockery not out of a plastic container.

Serves 4
Preparation time 5 minutes
Cooking time 20–30 minutes

Nutritional values
Calories 199
Kilojoules 835
Protein 15 g
Carbohydrates 1 g
Fat 14 g

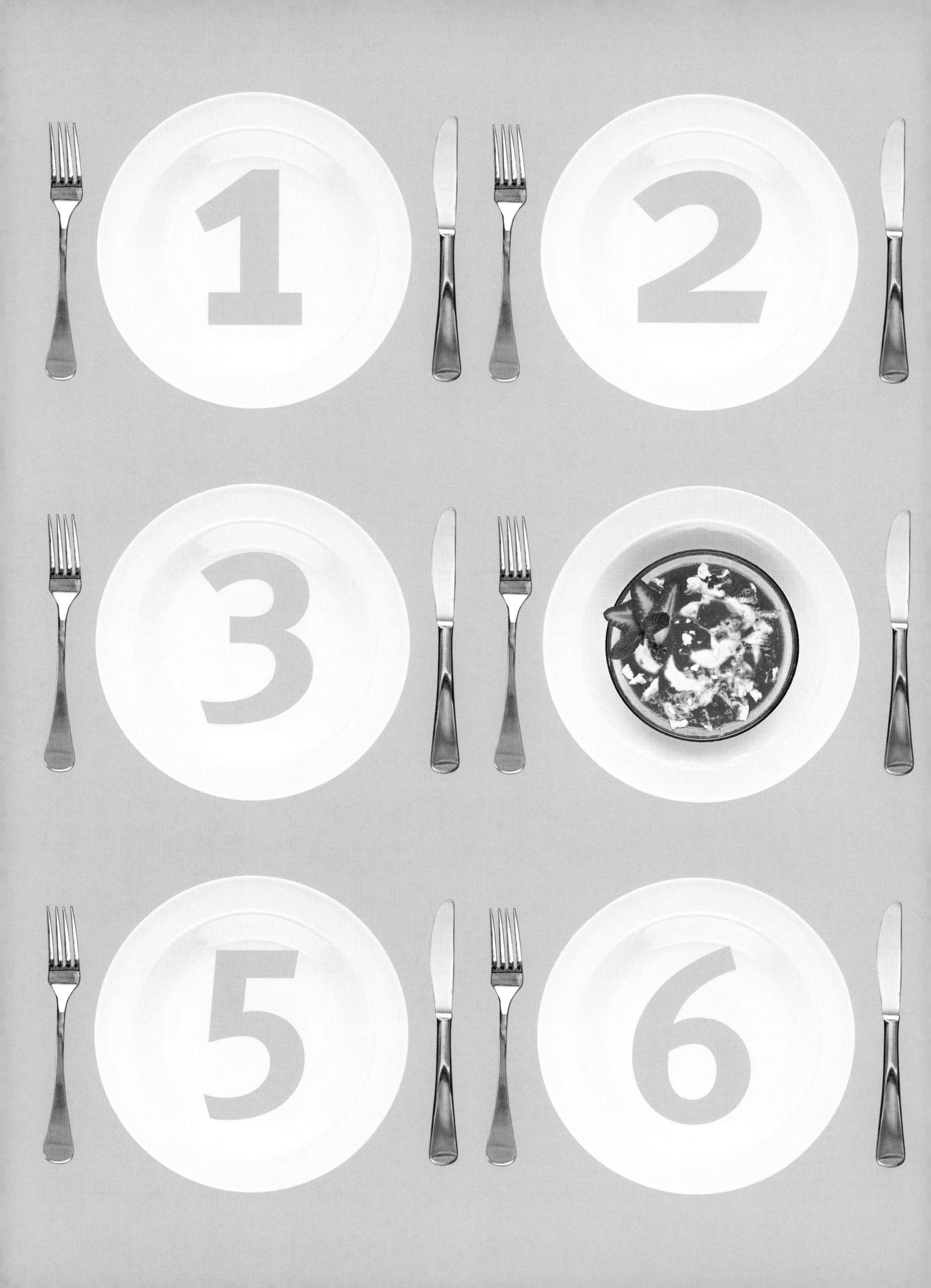
1
2
3
5
6

Afternoon snack

It is a very unusual person who doesn't once in a while feel the need for some kind of mid-afternoon pick-me-up. Dr Robert Thayer at California State University has determined that 4.34 p.m. precisely is when this is most likely to happen.

Our bodies take a natural dip in energy after lunch and unless we live in a Mediterranean country that encourages afternoon napping, we try to raise that energy by eating something sugary or caffeine-filled which produces an artificial energizing buzz. On top of this, the hormone serotonin, responsible for mood enhancement, dips mid-afternoon leaving us low in energy and enthusiasm. Carbohydrate foods help us make serotonin so our brain triggers us to crave them when it is low.

The snacks that we eat to fulfill our needs contain far greater amounts of carbohydrates (and the resultant calories) than we actually need. For example, you can boost serotonin with the amount of carbohydrate in one piece of toast and jelly (which weighs in at about 107 calories), but a more likely afternoon snack would be a jelly doughnut at 200+ calories. Also the amount of chocolate it takes to elevate mood is just four squares (around 1 oz) but the average candy bar actually weighs $2^1/_2$ oz. If you eat the whole bar rather than the simple squares of chocolate, then every day you will be eating roughly 166 chocolate-covered cheer-up calories (or 697 kj) you don't physically need to feel good — and creating a potential weight gain of 17 lb a year.

This doesn't mean that afternoon snacking should be discouraged. In fact, if you don't elevate your mood and energy now, you are more likely to be fed up when you get home at night where food is even more readily available to abuse. Plus, there's the simple biological fact that if you eat lunch at 1 p.m. and don't eat dinner until 6 or 7 p.m. you are going to be very hungry by the time you sit down to your evening meal and more likely to overeat. Because of this, afternoon snacking should be part of a healthy eating regime but it should include foods in the right quantities to avoid weight gain that actively create feelings of wellbeing.

Choose from 40 snacks

Like your morning snack, these treats contain around 100 calories a portion, but to satisfy potential sugar cravings and counteract that energy drop they are higher in carbohydrates, and are on the sweet side. You'll find a few treats like cookies that you might think shouldn't be on a diet plan. Don't eat these every day as they don't have great nutritional value, but do treat yourself on those days when you really feel you want them.

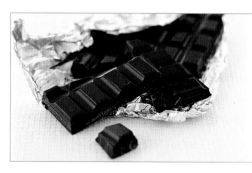

1 Four squares of good-quality (containing 70 percent or more of cocoa solids) **dark chocolate**.

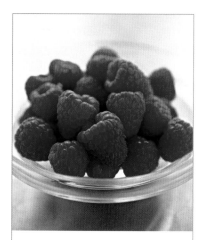

2 2 oz **dried apple**, mango, or banana chips.

3 One small slice of **jelly roll** (just under 1 inch thick).

6 2 tablespoons of **raspberries** served with half a honeydew melon.

4 One **crumpet** topped with a little low-fat spread.

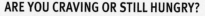

5 Any **granola bar** under 100 calories.

7 One small handful of unsalted **pretzels**.

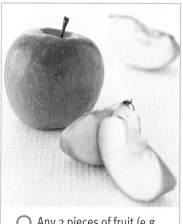

8 Any 2 pieces of fruit (e.g. **apple**, pear, or peach).

ARE YOU CRAVING OR STILL HUNGRY?

While people who weigh more than 180 lb may need more calories on this plan, if you have a very active job or exercise intensely you might also need to eat more to feel completely satisfied. One way to determine this, according to research published in the *International Journal of Eating Disorders*, is to look at what you crave in the afternoon; while sugary cravings are a cry for energy, salty cravings are a sign you need more nourishment.

If you crave salty foods such as peanut butter or popcorn in the afternoon but don't feel that you absolutely must have that item and that item alone (which is a sign of an emotional craving), perhaps you are not eating enough — especially if you have the traditional signs of hunger like a rumbling tummy or feeling light-headed. Try doubling the size of your morning snack, which will keep you fuller for longer, and if you still have problems add another large serving of vegetables or salad to any lunch. Exercisers should also take a look at the advice specifically for them on page 85.

If you have a bad morning, your afternoon snack cravings will be worse than normal. According to research from Penn State University in the US, many people, but particularly women, eat when the pressure is off rather than when they are stressed. If you feel this is happening to you, particularly good snack choices would be any choice containing blueberries, the Strawberry Crush recipe on page 84, or the choice of melon and raspberries. These are high in vitamin C, the presence of which causes stress hormones to fall more rapidly than normal, according to German research.

It will also do you good to take some time out after any stressful event to calm yourself down. Do this at your desk by pressing the acupressure point found between your thumb and forefinger, just at the base of the crease that forms when you press them together. Push this gently with your thumb and hold to relieve anxiety.

9 Four **Honey Balls** — mix 1 tablespoon of sesame seeds with 1 teaspoon of honey, form into balls and cool in the refrigerator for at least five minutes before eating.

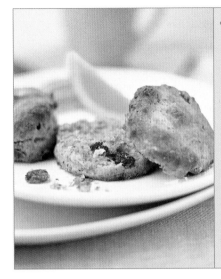

10 One **Orange and Raisin Scone** (see recipe on page 80) or half a small pre-made scone from the supermarket.

11 ¹/₂ cup low-fat **plain yogurt** mixed with 2 chopped, ready-to-eat dried apricots.

12 Two **oatcakes**, each topped with 1 teaspoon of low-sugar marmalade.

13 One small bag of low-fat **potato chips**, under 100 calories.

14 One small raisin **pancake** (around 1 ¹/₂ oz) topped with 1 teaspoon of honey.

15 One small handful (roughly 1 oz) of **yogurt-covered peanuts or raisins**.

16 Five **strawberries** dipped in 1 teaspoon of chocolate spread.

17 4 oz canned **fruit cocktail** in natural juice topped with 2 tablespoons of low-fat Greek or plain yogurt.

18 One **pear** halved and topped with 1 teaspoon of chocolate spread.

19 Two sticks of **celery** spread with 1 teaspoon of honey and topped with 2–3 raisins.

20 One handful of green or **red grapes** with 1 oz low-fat brie or Camembert cheese.

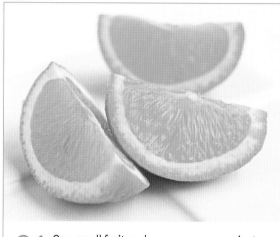

21 One small fruit such as an **orange**, apricot, plum, or kiwifruit with 1 fig roll biscuit.

SWIFT CRAVING SAPPERS

Got a sugar craving that won't quit even after you've eaten? Then sniff a little vanilla extract. Researchers at St George's Hospital, London, have found it stops sugar cravings almost instantly. If you find that you are suffering regularly, however, it might help to start taking a supplement of the herb rhodiola; this actively increases levels of serotonin in the brain, helps naturally balance blood sugar, and makes the body more resistant to stress, all of which help minimize many of the triggers for sugar cravings.

22 One slice of **fruit loaf** spread with a little low-fat cream cheese.

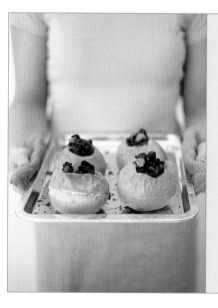

23 One **Fruity Baked Apple** (see recipe on page 83). If you don't have a sweet tooth, you can cut the calories on this recipe by leaving out the sugar.

24 Two **Melba toasts** topped with 2 tablespoons low-fat ricotta cheese and 1 teaspoon each of low-sugar jelly.

25 Ten small **gummy candies** like wine gums.

26 Three large **rice cakes** or 6 mini rice cakes, any flavor.

27 One sweet **waffle** topped with 1 teaspoon of apple sauce.

28 Individual pot of sugar-free **jello** served with a small carton of low-fat yogurt.

29 One **Orange Shortbread** (see recipe on page 87).

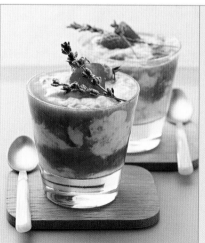

30 One serving of **Strawberry Crush** (see recipe on page 84). You could also try replacing the strawberries in this recipe with other berries such as raspberries or blueberries.

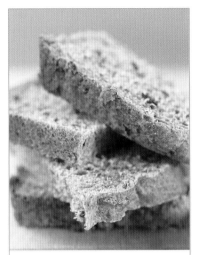

31 One slice of **wholegrain toast** topped with 1 teaspoon of honey or low-sugar jelly.

32 Five **prunes** — dried or canned in natural juice.

33 One slice of **Baked Almond and Apricot Cake** (see recipe on page 82).

34 Three **chocolate finger -style** cookies.

BREATHE YOURSELF THINNER

Most afternoon sugar cravings don't occur because you need candy; they happen to counteract the drop in energy that your brain experiences mid-afternoon. While nutritional means are the primary way to tackle this, they aren't the only energizing tactic you could use. Like everything in our body, lung function fluctuates throughout the day. But around noon and for a few hours afterwards it is at its lowest level. This makes you breathe more shallowly, increasing the levels of sedating carbon dioxide in your blood and decreasing the energizing oxygen.

A technique called belly breathing can counteract this. Sit up straight and breathe in deeply for a count of 5. As you do this, expand your stomach and try to fill your lungs right to the bottom. Now exhale for a count of 8–10 and contract your stomach back in to completely empty your lungs of all the stale air. Repeat until you feel more energized.

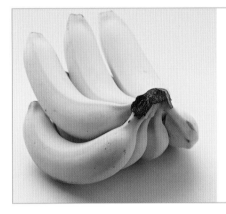

35 One small **banana** and 3 handfuls of blueberries, black currants, blackberries, or other soft fruit.

36 **Smoothie** made from 3/4 cup skim or soy milk blended with half a can of peaches canned in natural juice.

INSTANT FAT-SPOTTING

If you are in a meeting when afternoon snacktime hits, you can't break off to eat your prescribed snack, but you may able to sample some of the cookies offered. Relatively plain cookies like rich teas, fig bars, and ginger snaps, or old-fashioned cream cookies like custard creams or bourbons are around 50 calories each so two of these would be fine. Restrict yourself to only one chocolate-topped cookie or plain Graham cracker.

Cake is best avoided, unless there is a thin slice of angel cake or jelly roll on offer. If the cookies are homemade, a good test to determine their calories is to see just how much the cookie crumbles — the more crumbs it produces, the more fat it contains so only eat a few bites. The same goes for any cookies, cake, or muffin that leaves a greasy smudge when you put it on a napkin; this is a sign that it is high in fat so either leave it or just have two or three bites.

37 One small **fruit popsicle**.

38 One small pack (around 1^{1}/2 oz) **jelly beans**.

39 1 oz plain, unbuttered **popcorn**.

40 One **Rhubarb Bake** (see recipe on page 86).

Afternoon snack recipes

Preparing your own afternoon snacks helps ensure that you make the right choices at 3 p.m. instead of being swayed by high-fat treats. Many of the recipes here allow you to make batches of sweet treats in advance, ensuring you don't need to reach for whatever is available. If you find it hard to have sweet foods in the house without eating them, stick with individual serving snacks on the preceding pages.

Orange and raisin scones

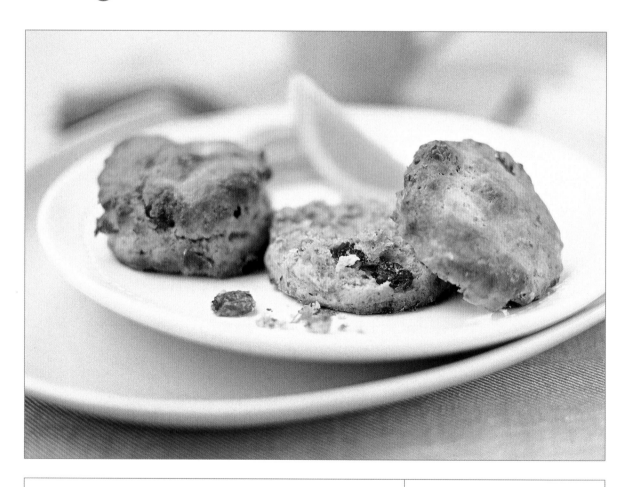

Makes 12
Preparation time 20 minutes
Cooking time about 10 minutes

Nutritional values
Calories 120
Kilojoules 505
Protein 3 g
Carbohydrates 18 g
Fat 4 g

1 cup self-rising flour, plus extra for dusting

1 cup wholewheat self-rising flour

2 teaspoons baking powder

$^1/_4$ cup butter, diced

$^1/_3$ cup golden raisins

1 tablespoon superfine sugar

grated zest of 1 orange

1 egg

about $^1/_2$ cup milk

1 Sift the flours and baking powder into a large bowl, tipping any bran in the sifter back into the bowl. Add the butter and blend with the fingertips until the mixture resembles fine bread crumbs, then stir in the golden raisins, sugar, and orange zest.

2 Break the egg into a measuring cup and beat it with a fork. Make up to $^2/_3$ cup with milk, pour into the flour mixture and bring together to form a soft dough, adding a little extra milk if the dough is too dry.

3 Press gently into a round, $^1/_2$ inch thick, and stamp out about 12 scones. Place them on lightly floured cookie sheets and brush with a little milk. Bake in a preheated oven, 425°F, for about 10 minutes or until risen and golden. Allow to cool on a wire rack. The scones can be stored in an airtight container for up to 3 days.

Citrus boosters

This recipe gives you a chance to use a generally ignored health booster — the zest of citrus fruits such as oranges, limes, and lemons. This part of the fruit contains ingredients called polymeth-oxylated flavones shown to lower cholesterol levels. It is also high in ingredients called d-limones which reduce the risk of skin cancer. Using zest in baking is probably the most palatable way to get the benefits — but if you are a fan of bitter foods you could also try sprinkling the grated zest over salads or mixing it into salsas.

Time for a siesta?

If you've been burning the candle at both ends, adding an afternoon nap to your weekend days can help boost the effects of your eating plan by fighting that post-lunch fatigue. But unless you want to feel worse when you wake up, keep naptime short. Researchers at Flinders University in South Australia found that ten minutes was the most refreshing amount of sleep. After this you go into a deep sleep, which, unless you complete the entire cycle (about 90 minutes) will leave you feeling groggy when you wake up. Longer sleeps can also sometimes interfere with your ability to get a good night's rest at the end of the day. So how do you know if you'll benefit from a nap? If it takes you less than ten minutes after getting into bed to fall asleep, you are overtired and need to catch up.

Baked almond and apricot cake

4 eggs

$^1/_2$ cup superfine sugar

$^1/_2$ teaspoon almond extract

$^1/_2$ cup all-purpose flour

$^3/_4$ cup ground almonds

APRICOT FILLING

$^3/_4$ cup ready-to-eat dried apricots

$^2/_3$–$^3/_4$ cup water

$^1/_2$ cup low-fat fromage frais or plain yogurt

1 Put the eggs, sugar, and almond extract in a large bowl and beat until thick and frothy. Sift the flour into the bowl and gently fold in with the ground almonds.

2 Line and lightly grease 2 round 7 inch baking pans. Divide the cake mixture between them. Bake in a preheated oven, 350°F, for 15–20 minutes. Allow to cool for 10 minutes then loosen the edges with a knife and turn out the layers onto a wire rack to cool.

3 To make the filling put the apricots in a small saucepan with the measured water, cover, and simmer for 10 minutes until softened. Puree in a blender or food processor until smooth.

4 Put one layer on a serving plate, spread with the cooled apricot purée and top with fromage frais or yogurt. Top with the second layer. Cut into 12 slices to serve. The cake can be stored in an airtight container for up to 3 days.

Sweeter when cooked

Baking fruit as you do in the recipe opposite changes the taste to something sweeter than when you eat it raw, especially if you integrate dried fruit in the recipe. If you are someone who doesn't think they like fruit, experimenting with cooked fruits like this can change your mind. Other techniques to try include broiling large slices of tropical fruits like pineapple or mango, or stewing fruits like plums or rhubarb with a teaspoon of sweetener.

Beware the danger days

While it might seem that weekends provide the easiest snacking possibilities, in fact, weekends are when you are most likely to skip your snacks. You are out and about and next thing you know it is dinnertime and you're starving. Good ways to remind yourself to snack are to set a watch alarm or just carry an easy snack like a granola bar in your bag so every time you reach in you are reminded that it is there.

Makes 12 slices
Preparation time 35 minutes
Cooking time 15–20 minutes

Nutritional values
Calories 122
Kilojoules 512
Protein 5 g
Carbohydrates 15 g
Fat 5 g

Fruity baked apple

4 large dessert apples

4 oz ready-to-eat dried fruit (such as cranberries, golden raisins and apricots)

4 teaspoons raw sugar

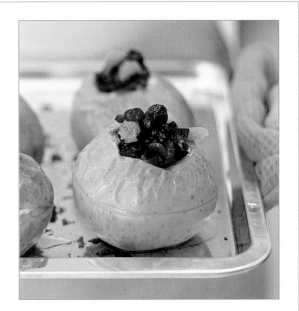

1 Core the apples and score a line around the middle of the fruit and arrange them in an ovenproof dish. Stuff the cored center of the apples with the dried fruit.

2 Sprinkle with the sugar and bake in a preheated oven, 400°F, for 25 minutes or until the apples are tender. Cut in half and serve.

Serves 4
Preparation time 5 minutes
Cooking time 25 minutes

Nutritional values
Calories 127
Kilojoules 533
Protein 1 g
Carbohydrates 32 g
Fat 0 g

Strawberry crush

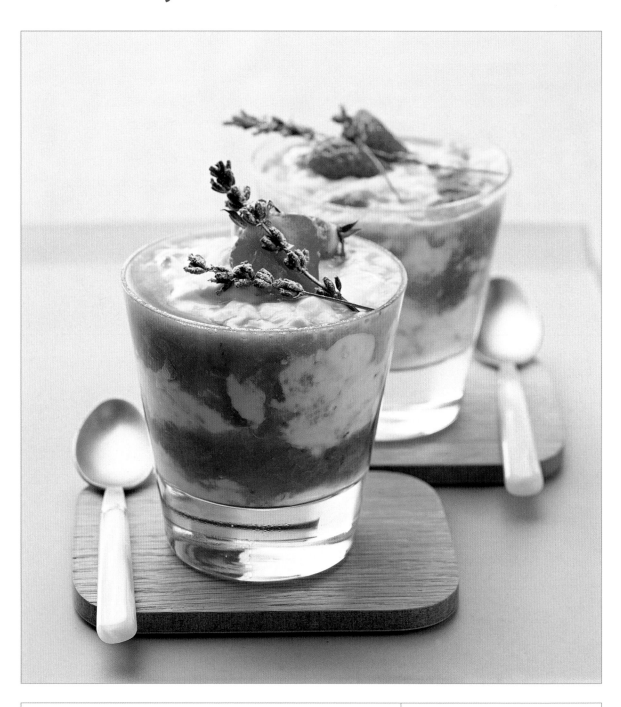

Serves 4
Preparation time 5 minutes

Nutritional values
Calories 122
Kilojoules 512
Protein 7 g
Carbohydrates 23 g
Fat 0 g

2^1/$_2$ cups strawberries, washed and hulled

1 tablespoon confectioners' sugar

1^1/$_4$ cups low-fat fromage frais or plain yogurt

4 ready-made meringue nests

1 Mash the strawberries with the confectioners' sugar using a fork or food processor.

2 Put the fromage frais or yogurt in a bowl, crumble in the meringues and mix together lightly.

3 Add the strawberry mixture and fold together with a spoon until marbled. Spoon into glasses and serve with a sprig of lavender (optional).

High GI?

This dish might look like a recipe for post-sugar hunger pangs as meringue is a very high GI food that converts quickly to sugar in the body. However, strawberries and fromage frais are low GI foods, so adding them slows down the speed at which this dish is digested. You can cut the calories (and the GI) further by taking out the sugar and adding another ^{1}/$_3$ cup strawberries, which will also boost your intake of vitamin C.

Are you an evening exerciser?

Physiologically, after work is the best time for our body to exercise — our muscles are at their warmest and people generally say exercise feels easier at this point. To make the most of this biological boost, the snack you choose mid-afternoon is very important as it will fuel your workout. Choosing the lower glycemic snacks from the choices here — oatcakes, the pear with chocolate spread or yogurt and apricots — is a good start, but if you are exercising intensely (running, cycling, or doing a high-intensity aerobics class like step or spinning) for more than 45 minutes, you may want to double the calories you consume for your afternoon snack. You can do this by combining any two snacks suggested here, doubling the serving size or adding a little low-fat dairy product like a small 4 oz carton of low-fat fruit yogurt or fromage frais.

Rhubarb bakes

¹/₄ cup margarine

2 tablespoons corn syrup

1 tablespoon light brown sugar

³/₄ cup rolled oats

¹/₂ cup wholewheat self-rising flour, sifted

pinch of ground ginger

¹/₄ cup pecan nuts, chopped

6 tablespoons rhubarb compote or stewed rhubarb

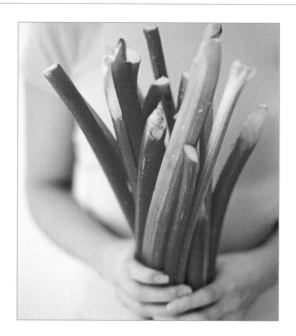

1 Place the margarine, syrup, and sugar in a pan and heat gently until the sugar is dissolved. Stir in the oats, flour, ginger, and nuts and combine well.

2 Spoon two-thirds of the mixture into a 6 inch square, nonstick baking pan and gently press down. Spoon over the rhubarb, sprinkle over the remaining oat mixture and press down lightly.

3 Bake in a preheated oven, 350°F, for 15 minutes until golden. Cool in the pan, marking the mixture into 8 rectangles while still warm.

Makes 8
Preparation time 10 minutes
Cooking time 15 minutes

Nutritional values
Calories 120
Kilojoules 504
Protein 2 g
Carbohydrates 12 g
Fat 5 g

Orange shortbread

$^1/_2$ cup all-purpose flour

3 tablespoons unsalted butter, diced

grated zest of $^1/_4$ orange

pinch of mixed spice

$1^1/_2$ tablespoons superfine sugar

$^1/_2$ teaspoon cold water

1 Sift the flour into a bowl, add the butter and blend with the fingertips until the mixture resembles fine bread crumbs. Stir in the remaining ingredients with the water and combine to form a ball.

2 Roll out on a lightly floured surface to $^1/_8$ inch thick. Use a $2^1/_2$ inch cutter to cut out about 6 rounds.

3 Place the rounds on a nonstick cookie sheet and bake in a preheated oven, 400°F, for 10–12 minutes until golden. Transfer to a wire rack and allow to cool. The shortbread can be stored in an airtight container for up to 5 days.

When afternoon carbs might not work for you

If you want your afternoon energy boost to be primarily mental not physical, you can skip the sugary treats and choose a suggestion from one of the morning snacks on offer. While serotonin makes us feel good, it is also a sedating and calming hormone — for intense mental function you'll do better producing dopamine in your body which increases alertness, concentration, and reaction times and you get this by eating protein foods.

Remember to eat less

If you are used to having a sugary treat like a sticky bun or candy bar in the afternoon, use this simple psychological trick to ensure that you feel satisfied with the smaller treats suggested. Remember exactly what you ate for breakfast, lunch, and your mid-morning snack and remember how full and satisfied you felt after each meal. According to research at the University of Birmingham in the UK, when people did this they naturally ate a much smaller than normal afternoon snack and felt satisfied with it.

Makes 6
Preparation time 10 minutes
Cooking time 10–12 minutes

Nutritional values
Calories 95
Kilojoules 399
Protein 1 g
Carbohydrates 10 g
Fat 6 g

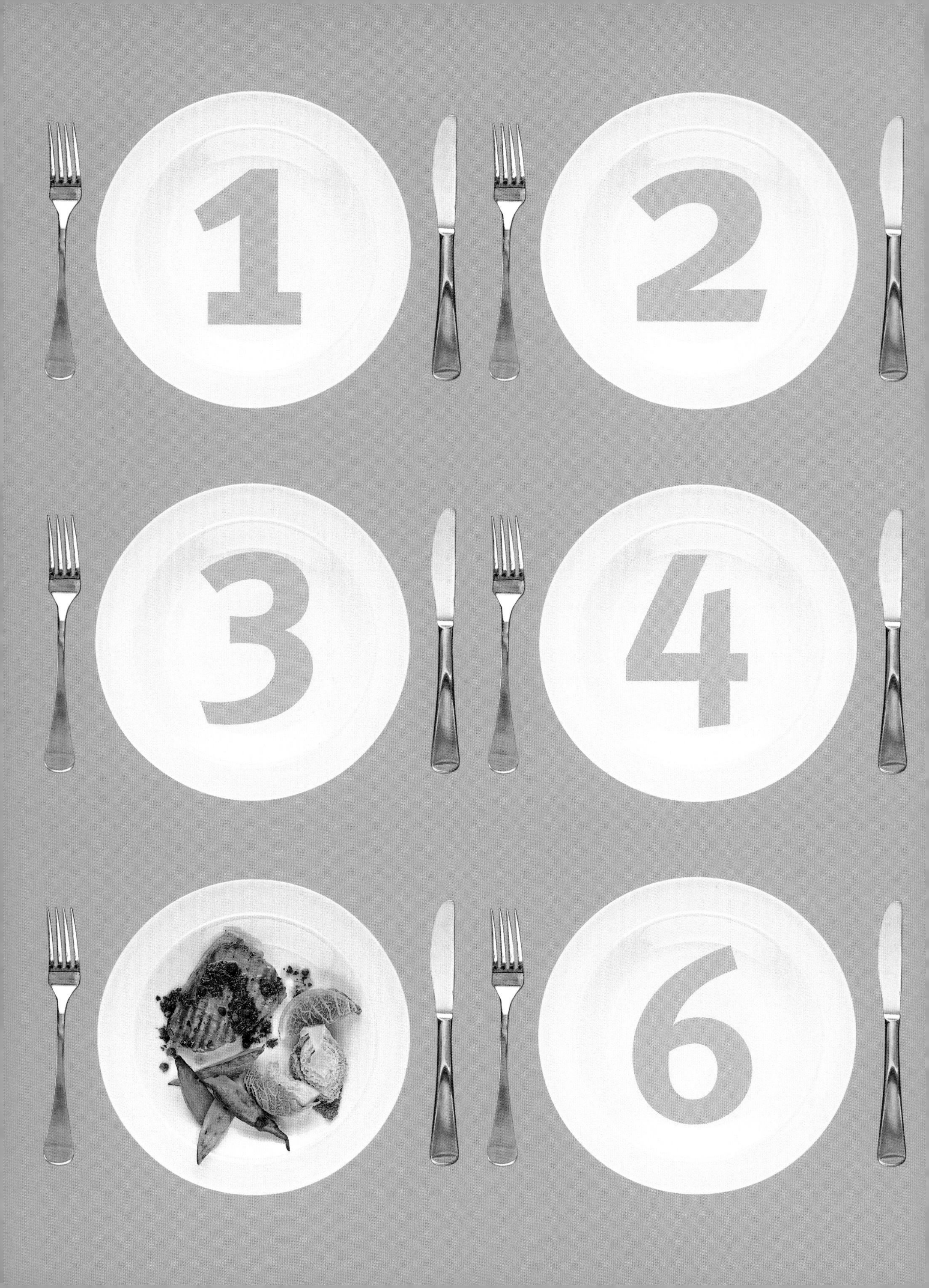
1
2
3
4
6

Dinner

In recent years there has been a fad for diets to focus on lighter evening meals
— either by cutting out whole food groups (most commonly carbohydrates) or by
allowing you to eat those carbs but only before, say, 6 p.m. The theory is that if
you eat too many calories or large amounts of carbohydrates in the evening, your
body won't be able to burn them off, so that they are more likely to be stored as fat.
It's a good theory, but it doesn't seem to be true.

According to a study of 1800 women by the City University in New York,
the time of day women ate their calories was irrelevant to weight gain
— how many calories they ate determined whether the needle on the
scales went up or down. And even more conclusively, a study of 7000
women found that even if they ate 50 percent of their calories after
5 p. m., they were no more likely to gain weight than those who ate half
that amount at the day's end. In fact, given the research discussed on
page 21 that explained how calories actually become less satisfying by
the end of the day, it makes sense to eat a slightly larger dinner at
night so you feel full and eliminate the need to nibble.

But the key word here is "slightly"; the average body burns about
60 calories an hour lying around doing nothing (the way many of us
spend our evenings before we retire to bed). Therefore, whereas a
meal of 700 or more calories may not be completely used up before
you eat again, a meal of 400–500 calories will easily be burnt up
between the time you eat it (ideally at 6–7.30 p.m.) and breakfast time
the next morning at 6–8 a.m. Even accounting for the extra calories
from the bedtime snack you will read about in the next chapter and the
slight decline in metabolic rate overnight, you will still be unlikely to
eat more calories than you can burn if you keep your meal size
moderate. Because of this, the evening meals suggested in this plan fit
into that 400–500 calorie span. While they are moderate in calories,
they are satisfyingly full of all the nutrients your body needs to carry
out its nightly regeneration and repair.

Choose from 50 dinners

Evening is when most of us prefer to have our biggest meal. Time for its preparation is generally limited (except for weekends) which is why virtually all the meals here are quick and easy to prepare, and will work both for you and any non-dieting members of your family. No more picking at a salad while the rest of the family tuck in. You can serve these dishes to everyone.

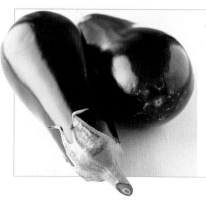

1 One **eggplant** halved and roasted in the oven with a little olive oil until soft. Top with 1 oz feta cheese thinly sliced, 2 tablespoons grated low-fat cheddar, and $^1/_4$ cup pine nuts. Broil until the cheese bubbles. Serve with $^1/_4$ cup pilau rice.

2 **Stir-fry** 4 oz firm tofu and 2 tablespoons cashew nuts plus unlimited snowpeas, baby corn, and red bell pepper in 2 teaspoons of sesame oil, a little chili, and some soy sauce. Serve with 2 oz dry weight of egg noodles.

3 $3^1/_2$ oz **squid rings** in batter, broiled. Serve with $^1/_4$ cup brown rice, a dab of sweet chili sauce, and a small green salad.

4 **Bolognaise sauce** made from 3 oz lean ground beef, turkey, or meat-substitute protein, 2–3 handfuls of mushrooms and 1 cup prepared tomato sauce served on 2 oz pasta.

TURN OFF YOUR TV TO GET THIN

It is estimated that every two hours of TV watching increases your risk of obesity by 23 percent. One reason is that television actively slows down your metabolic rate; according to researchers at Tulane University in the US you burn 20–30 calories an hour less watching television than you would lying completely still. Plus the constant presence of food advertising within commercials can tempt you into snack attacks.

Try to keep at least two nights a week television free on this plan and do something more active or at least actively relaxing instead. If you do want to keep up with the soaps and keep your weight down, at least spend commercial breaks doing a few simple exercises like sit-ups or squats or walking up and down stairs. If you watch two one-hour programs a night, but walk stairs during each advertising break, you'd actually do 20 minutes of stair-climbing a night.

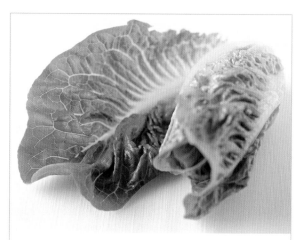

5 **Caesar-style salad** made from unlimited lettuce topped with 2 tablespoons low-fat Caesar dressing, $^1/_3$ cup grated Parmesan cheese and 1 oz croutons. Top with 4 oz broiled chicken or new potatoes and 1 sliced boiled egg.

6 One **spinach and ricotta cannelloni ready meal** (around 350 calories) served with a side salad of spinach, red bell peppers, and $1/4$ cup pumpkin seeds or pine nuts.

7 4 oz **lamb chop** (all fat removed) served with 1 cup lima beans mashed with 2 teaspoons of low-fat sour cream and served with 1 corn ear.

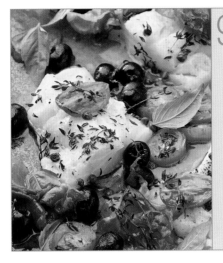

9 One serving of **Roasted Cod with Prosciutto** (see recipe on page 96) served with 5 oz new potatoes and unlimited green beans, or any other green vegetable steamed or boiled.

8 Half a **foccacia or ciabatta** loaf (around 4 oz) topped with 3 tablespoons of low-fat hummus and broiled slices of red and yellow bell pepper. Serve with a salad of lettuce leaves topped with balsamic vinegar and a few olives.

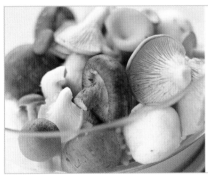

10 One serving of **Mushroom Stroganoff** (see recipe on page 99) served with 3 oz brown rice or pasta shapes and a large green salad.

11 5 oz serving of **chicken tikka fillets** (from supermarket) served with a 7 oz selection of mixed vegetables (carrot, green beans, mushrooms, and onion) cooked with 3 tablespoons of ready-made curry sauce and 2 microwaved pappadoms.

12 Any low-fat **ready meal** under 400 calories served with unlimited vegetables.

13 One fillet of **cod** in bread crumbs served with 4 oz potato wedges and 3 tablespoons of coleslaw.

14 4 oz lean **steak,** broiled and served with 5 oz new potatoes, 2 broiled tomatoes and unlimited green beans.

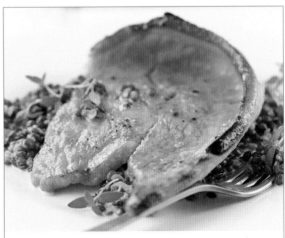

15 5 oz **salmon fillet** served with 4 oz potato salad, either store-bought or made with boiled potatoes mixed with a little low-fat mayonnaise and red onion, and unlimited asparagus.

16 5 oz **ham steak** served with 8 oz canned lentils or $1/3$ cup red lentils cooked as directed. Serve with unlimited green beans.

TRY TO DO SOMETHING DIFFERENT

Many of us have evening habits that we associate with eating — you might get home, switch on the news, and have a glass of wine to wind down. Or you always walk home past a fast-food restaurant and if you're too tired to cook you generally stop by. If you videotaped the news and had a bath to wind down instead, or you didn't walk past that fast-food place, you wouldn't be tempted to drink the wine or buy the fast food.

Changing behaviors like this are the key to an approach called the "Do Something Different" plan, and volunteers at the UK University of Hertfordshire trial lost 11 lb in four months without actively dieting — think what you could change about your evening routine to power up your weight loss and boost your results.

17 4 oz **roast lamb** (all fat removed) served with unlimited red or green cabbage, 5 oz new potatoes, and 1 tablespoon of gravy.

18 One serving of **Moussaka** (see recipe on page 107) served with a salad of lettuce, red bell pepper, and $1/4$ avocado.

19 5 oz **sole fillet**, broiled and topped with a little lemon juice. Serve with a selection of vegetables including unlimited bell peppers, eggplant, onion, and 3 diced sweet potatoes roasted until soft with 1 tablespoon olive oil and some fresh herbs.

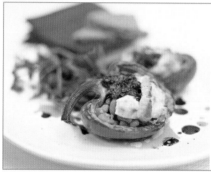

20 One serving of **Grilled Peppers with Goats Cheese** (see recipe on page 102) served with a green salad and 3 small slices of garlic bread.

21 **Omelet** made with 2 whole eggs and filled with 3 slices of lean ham or unlimited mushrooms, plus $1/4$ cup grated cheese. Serve with unlimited broiled zucchini.

22 **Shepherd's pie** made with 3 oz lean ground beef or 4 oz soy meat substitute mixed with chopped carrots, onion, and 2 tablespoons of gravy and topped with 5 oz mashed potato. Serve with unlimited Savoy cabbage.

23 **Pizza** made from 1 individual ready-made pizza base (around 3 oz) spread with 1 tablespoon tomato paste and topped with 4 slices of prosciutto and/or 5 sliced artichoke hearts and 4 sliced mushrooms. Sprinkle over 2 oz low-fat mozzarella, grated. Serve with a large green salad.

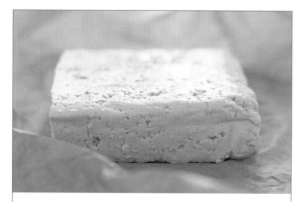

24 4 oz **tofu or shrimp** stir-fried with unlimited vegetables and 4 tablespoons of prepared sweet and sour sauce. Serve on $1/4$ cup brown rice.

25 4 oz lean **steak** cut into strips or 2 oz canned kidney beans stir-fried with slices of red and yellow bell pepper and chili powder to taste. Serve inside two tortilla wraps spread with half an avocado, mashed, and some salsa.

26 Two **fresh sardines**, broiled and served with $1/3$ cup couscous and a large tomato and onion salad.

27 Two low-fat or vegetarian **sausages** served with 5 oz potatoes mashed with a little skim milk and some salt. Serve with $1/2$ cup peas.

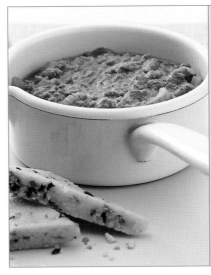

28 One serving of **Beef ragout with Polenta Wedges** (see recipe on page 100). You can replace the polenta in this recipe with a fist-sized chunk of crusty wholegrain bread if you prefer.

SIT UP STRAIGHT

Research from the University of Adelaide in Australia has reported that you feel less full after eating slumped on the sofa than if you eat upright at a table. If you tend toward TV dinners, make a switch to table eating, and if you don't have a dining table, at least sit up straight on the sofa to eat.

29 Two large flat-topped **mushrooms,** broiled and topped with a mixture of 4 chopped walnuts and 2 oz crumbled Stilton cheese. Serve with $1/3$ cup couscous and unlimited spinach.

30 One low-fat quarter-pounder **hamburger** or vegetarian burger broiled and served with 5 oz low-fat oven fries. Serve with 2 tablespoons of salsa and 3 tablespoons of coleslaw.

31 One meat-substitute protein **steak** served with a 7 oz baked potato topped with 7 oz ratatouille.

32 One serving of **Pork Scallops with Lemon and Capers** (see recipe on page 98) served with 2 small roasted sweet potatoes and unlimited Savoy cabbage.

33 One **Chicken Burger with Tomato Salsa** (see recipe on page 103) or a large vegetarian burger served in a burger bun with a side salad of lettuce, cucumber, and $1/2$ an avocado, sliced.

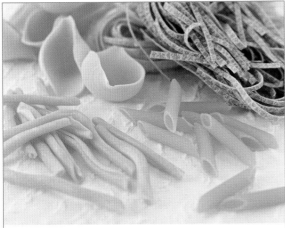

34 **Pasta** dish of 2 Canadian or vegetarian bacon slices broiled until crispy, chopped, and added to 7 oz serving of any ready-made mushroom pasta sauce and combined with 2 oz pasta shells.

35 **Kebabs** made from skewered cubes of bell pepper, onion, and mushrooms with 4 oz smoked tofu or a firm fish like angler fish, broiled. Serve with a 7 oz baked potato and 2 tablespoons of sweet chili sauce.

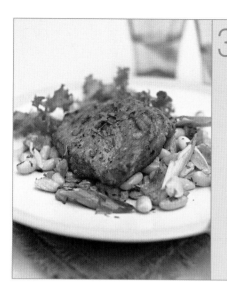

36 One serving of **Liver with Leeks and Cannellini Beans** (see recipe on page 106) served with 1 small slice of focaccia or ciabatta bread. If you don't like liver, the recipe works as well with the same sized portion of steak or a pork chop.

37 Four **fish sticks** served with 5 oz oven fries and 5 oz low-sugar baked beans.

38 5 oz **chicken breast** served with 3 medium roasted potatoes and unlimited cabbage.

39 One ready-made **Chicken Kiev** served with unlimited broccoli and peas.

40 One large 8 oz **baked potato**. Top with 4 oz canned tuna in brine mixed with a little low-fat mayonnaise and serve with 7 oz ratatouille.

41 **Feta cheese salad** of unlimited arugula topped with 6 sun-dried tomatoes, 1 oz feta cheese and $1/4$ avocado, sliced. Top with 4 oz broiled shrimp or serve with 2 small slices of garlic bread.

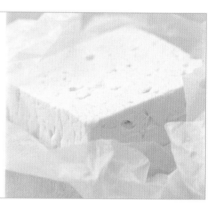

42 2 oz **pasta** shapes mixed with 2 tablespoons of fresh pesto sauce. Serve with a large salad of sliced tomato and red onion.

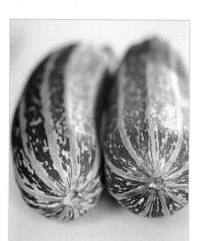

43 Half a **vegetable marrow**, cored then stuffed with a mix of 2 oz dry weight sage and onion stuffing and 2 tablespoons pine nuts. Roast until soft. Serve with 4 oz mashed potatoes, unlimited carrots, and 1 tablespoon of gravy.

QUICK QUESTION

I often don't get in from work until 9 p.m. and I'm too tired to cook. What should I do?

Firstly, add an extra snack into your diet about 6.30 p.m. This will replace your before-bed snack, but will keep your metabolism from falling between your mid-afternoon eating and when you finally do get time to eat. You can choose from either the morning or afternoon snack for this, but do remember that the protein-based morning snack will give greater levels of satiety and a higher metabolic boost.

Then, either choose the option above that allows you to have any ready meal with a mixed salad or just serve yourself $2/3$ cup of any breakfast cereal with $3/4$ cup of skim milk and any two pieces of fruit. It's a slightly lower calorie meal than the evening options suggested here, but it is packed with nutrients.

44 1^{1}/$_{2}$ cups of any fresh carton **soup**. Serve with half a ciabatta loaf (around 4 oz) spread with a thin layer of baba ganoush. Top with slices of broiled zucchini.

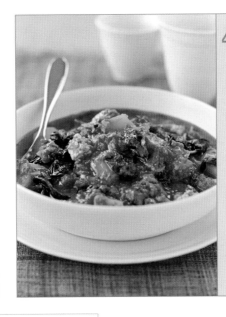

45 One serving of **Tempeh Balti** (see recipe on page 104) served with 1 mini (around 2 oz) naan bread, 2 microwave pappadums with a dab of lime pickle or 2 tablespoons dry weight basmati rice.

46 5 oz **salmon fillet** topped with a sauce made from 1^{1}/$_{2}$ oz watercress pureed with ^{1}/$_{2}$ cup low-fat plain yogurt. Serve with 5 oz new potatoes and unlimited broccoli.

47 One **Mediterranean flatbread** spread with ^{1}/$_{2}$ teaspoon of harissa paste and 1 tablespoon of tsatziki. Fill with 3 oz sliced roast lamb or 2 sliced portobello mushrooms and 2 tablespoons pine nuts and a little diced cucumber and tomato. Serve with ^{1}/$_{3}$ cup couscous.

48 Two **crunchy taco shells** filled with chili made from 4 oz ground turkey or soy meat substitute and 2 oz of canned kidney beans, 7 oz canned tomatoes and ^{1}/$_{2}$ teaspoon of chili powder. Serve with ^{1}/$_{2}$ avocado, sliced.

49 4 oz **trout fillet** or fresh tuna steak, broiled with a little lemon and served with ^{1}/$_{2}$ cup brown rice and unlimited green beans.

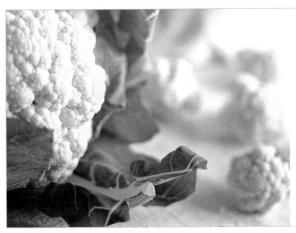

50 **Cauliflower cheese** made from unlimited cauliflower topped with a sauce made from 1 tablespoon melted butter, add 1 heap teaspoon of flour and mix well. Add ^{2}/$_{3}$ cup skim milk and 1 oz low-fat cheddar, keep stirring until the sauce thickens. Serve with a large green salad and 2 slices of garlic bread.

Dinner recipes

If there is one point in the day when most of us make an effort with our meal it is evening time, but making an effort doesn't need to mean slaving over a hot stove for hours. The recipes here, while tasty enough to grace any dinner party, are also quick and easy enough to fit into most busy lives even just once a week. If you're starting to get bored on the plan, don't quit; instead take the time one evening to try one of these dishes to reinforce the idea that losing weight needn't be a trial.

Roasted cod with prosciutto

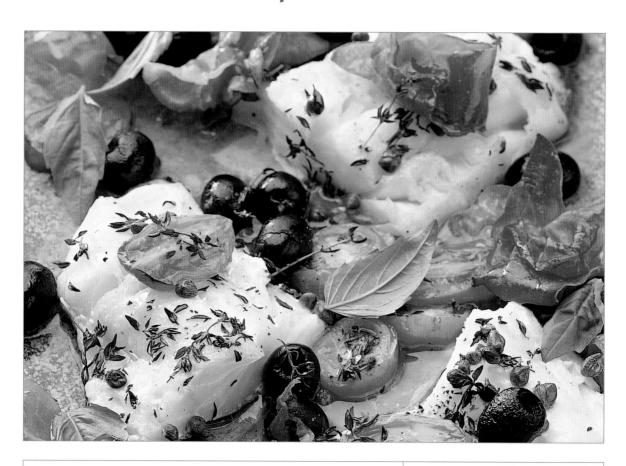

Serves 4
Preparation time 2 minutes
Cooking time 15 minutes

Nutritional values
Calories 349
Kilojoules 1466
Protein 35 g
Carbohydrates 7 g
Fat 22 g

12 oz cherry tomatoes, halved

1/3 cup pitted black olives

2 tablespoons capers, drained and rinsed

grated zest and juice of 1 lemon

2 teaspoons chopped thyme

4 tablespoons extra virgin olive oil

4 cod fillets, about 6 oz each

4 slices of prosciutto

salt and pepper

1 Combine the tomatoes, olives, capers, lemon zest, thyme, and oil in a roasting pan and season with salt and pepper.

2 Fit the cod fillets in the pan, spooning some of the tomato mixture over the fish. Scatter the prosciutto over the top and roast in a preheated oven, 425°F, for 15 minutes.

3 Remove the pan from the oven, drizzle over the lemon juice, cover with foil and allow to rest for 5 minutes before serving.

Fabulous fish

Ounce for ounce, fish contains far less calories than meat and is a great source of metabolism-boosting protein. According to studies published in the prestigious *British Medical Journal*, the average fish-eater weighs 7 lb less than those who eat mainly meat. On top of this, fish-eaters have less risk of depression, fewer cases of asthma, and a lowered risk of many cancers. It is recommended that most people eat at least two servings of fish a week, including one of oily fish like salmon, sardines, or mackerel.

Time for some fast food

You'll notice that all the evening meals suggested here are home-cooked (or at least bought from a supermarket). There is a reason for this — the average person who eats out more than five times a week consumes an average of 300 calories more than a home-cooker each day. However, this doesn't mean that one night a week, if you really want it, you can't have a fast-food meal on this diet plan. Remember, you have 500 calories to play with. You could have:
• A standard serving of beef/chicken/seafood in oyster or black bean sauce or stir-fried with vegetables and 3 tablespoons boiled rice.
• One small-sized portion of Tandoori Chicken or Chicken Tikka with 3 tablespoons of rice, dahl, or vegetable curry.
• Small-sized portion of any seafood or tomato-based pasta with 2 small slices of garlic bread.

Pork scallops with lemon and capers

1 tablespoon chopped flat leaf parsley

3 tablespoons chopped mint

4–6 tablespoons lemon juice

1 tablespoon capers, drained and rinsed

6 tablespoons olive oil, plus extra for brushing

4 pork scallops, each about 4 oz, trimmed

1 Place the herbs, lemon juice, capers, and olive oil in a blender and puree until smooth to make a dressing.

2 Brush the pork with olive oil and place the scallops on a preheated hot griddle pan. Cook for 2–3 minutes on each side or until cooked through.

3 Drizzle the lemon and caper dressing over the pork and serve immediately.

Are you hungry or just fed up?

Evenings are prime-time for emotional eating binges where you use food to cheer yourself up after a bad day. A key sign that this is what's happening to you is a craving for one particular food that hits suddenly. If you suffer from this, having non-food treats around is a key way to beat the syndrome. Stock up with one or more of the following and use these to take your mind off food when comfort eating strikes.
• A delicious-smelling bubble bath.
• The box set of your favorite TV show or movie on DVD.
• A new book or magazine that keeps you engaged.
• A solitaire or sports game on the computer.
• A set of proper stationery to write to friends.
• A list of movie times pinned to the refrigerator so you can take yourself out of "harm's way."

Serves 4
Preparation time 15 minutes
Cooking time 10 minutes

Nutritional values
Calories 401
Kilojoules 1684
Protein 46 g
Carbohydrates 0 g
Fat 28 g

Mushroom stroganoff

1 tablespoon canola oil

1 large onion, thinly sliced

4 celery sticks, thinly sliced

2 garlic cloves, crushed

1$^1/_4$ lb mixed mushrooms, roughly chopped

2 teaspoons smoked paprika

1 cup vegetable stock

$^2/_3$ cup sour cream

pepper

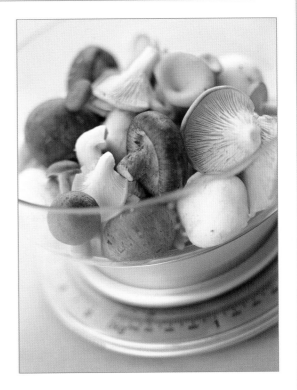

1 Heat the oil in a nonstick skillet and cook the onion, celery, and garlic for 5 minutes or until beginning to soften. Add the mushrooms and paprika and cook for a further 5 minutes.

2 Pour in the stock and cook for an additional 10 minutes or until the liquid is reduced by half.

3 Stir in the sour cream and season with pepper to taste. Cook over a medium heat for 5 minutes. Serve immediately.

Serves 4
Preparation time 10 minutes
Cooking time 25 minutes

Nutritional values
Calories 90
Kilojoules 378
Protein 27 g
Carbohydrates 7 g
Fat 14 g

Beef ragout with polenta wedges

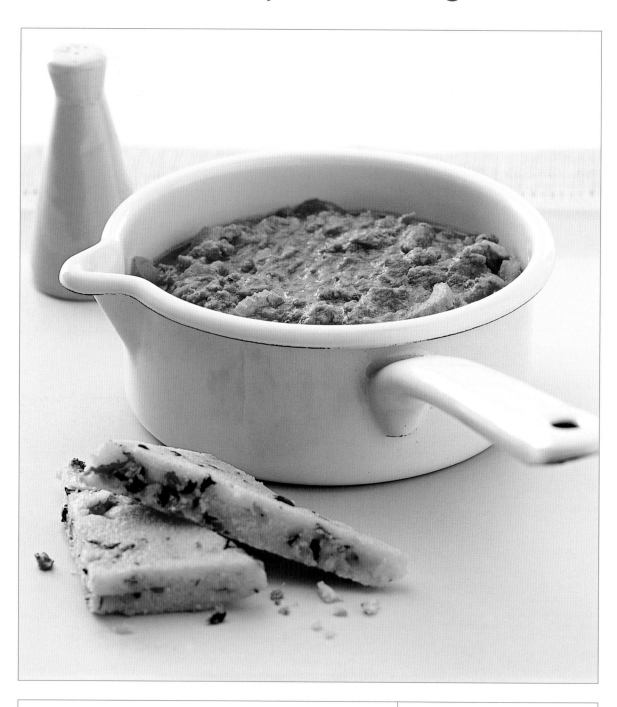

Serves 4
Preparation time 15 minutes
Cooking time 40 minutes

Nutritional values
Calories 520
Kilojoules 2184
Protein 38 g
Carbohydrates 42 g
Fat 25 g

vegetable oil, for cooking

1 red onion, finely chopped

1 garlic clove, chopped

2 celery sticks, chopped

1 lb lean ground beef

2 x 13 oz cans chopped tomatoes

$1/4$ cup tomato paste

$3/4$ cup red wine

1 teaspoon dried mixed herbs

pepper

WEDGES

1 cup quick-cook cornmeal

$3/4$ cup freshly grated Parmesan cheese

2 oz sun-dried tomatoes (not in oil), roughly chopped

$1/3$ cup pitted black olives, drained, rinsed, and roughly chopped

1 teaspoon roughly chopped rosemary

1 Lightly oil a large, nonstick saucepan, heat the pan and cook the onion, garlic, and celery for 5 minutes. Add the ground beef and cook over a medium heat until browned. Stir in the tomatoes, tomato paste, red wine, herbs, and pepper. Bring to a boil, then reduce the heat and simmer for 30 minutes or until the liquid has reduced by about half.

2 Make the polenta wedges. Bring $2^1/2$ cups water to a boil in a large saucepan. Slowly pour in the cornmeal, stirring continually. Reduce the heat to low and cook for 1 minute. Stir in the Parmesan, sun-dried tomatoes, olives, and rosemary and season to taste with pepper. Spread the polenta in a lightly oiled, 7–11 inch shallow pan. Allow to cool, then cut into 16 triangles.

3 Place the polenta under a preheated hot broiler for 3–4 minutes. Transfer to a warm plate and serve with the beef

Just desserts?

If you are used to having dessert right after dinner, you are going to be craving sweet foods practically as soon as you put down your fork. To stop the craving in its tracks, head to the bathroom and clean your teeth — the mint taste will overpower your tastebuds, helping them to forget the craving.

Oil spray

Every tablespoon of oil you cook with in a recipe adds 100 calories (420 kj) and roughly 14 g of fat to your daily intake; if you switch to an oil spray for tasks like frying spices, to moisten meats such as steak that you want to brown or completely for dishes such as stir-fries, you will only use around 2 calories (0.5 kj) a spritz. You'll find oil sprays in most supermarkets or to make your own, buy a garden sprayer (like the ones you use to mist plants) and fill it with 1 part oil to 7 parts water.

Grilled peppers with goat cheese

4 red bell peppers, halved, cored, and seeded

13 oz canned flageolet beans, drained
  and rinsed

4 teaspoons olive oil

4 oz firm goat cheese

8 teaspoons ready-made pesto

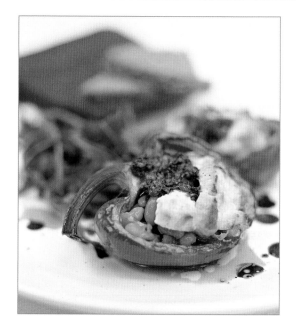

1 Put the pepper halves on a baking sheet, skin
  side down, and divide the flageolet beans
among them. Drizzle with the oil.

2 Cut the goat cheese horizontally into 2 slices
  and arrange them on top of the peppers. Top
each one with 1 teaspoon pesto.

3 Cover the peppers with foil and bake in a
  preheated oven, 400°F, for 20 minutes or until
the peppers are tender. Remove the foil and bake for
an additional 10 minutes.

Serves 4
Preparation time 5 minutes
Cooking time 30 minutes

Nutritional values
Calories 350
Kilojoules 1470
Protein 17 g
Carbohydrates 47 g
Fat 12 g

Chicken burgers with tomato salsa

BURGERS

1 garlic clove, crushed

3 scallions, finely sliced

1 tablespoon ready-made pesto

2 tablespoons fresh mixed herbs (such as parsley, tarragon, and thyme)

12 oz ground chicken

2 sun-dried tomatoes, finely chopped

1 teaspoon olive oil

TOMATO SALSA

8 oz cherry tomatoes, quartered

1 red chili, cored, seeded, and finely chopped

1 tablespoon chopped cilantro

grated zest and juice of 1 lime

1 Mix together all the ingredients for the burgers except the oil. Divide the mixture into 4 and form neat, flattened rounds. Chill for 30 minutes.

2 Meanwhile, combine all the tomato salsa ingredients together in a bowl.

3 Lightly brush the burgers with oil and cook under a preheated hot broiler or on a barbecue for 3–4 minutes each side until cooked through. Serve immediately with the salsa.

Warning — hidden calories in sight

Cooking and clearing-up time can be prime danger points for consuming unnoticed calories — tasting sauces while you cook, eating that bit of cheese that's too small to put back in the refrigerator or eating the bits of fish sticks or burger left by the children as you clear away their plates. One way to avoid these calories is to wear disposable gloves while you cook or clear up (obviously taking them off if you're doing any kind of kneading or hand mixing). Because they feel odd against your tongue you'll notice as you put your hands to your mouth and can stop yourself from nibbling without realizing. Chewing gum also works, as does carrying a pot of salt with you as you clear leftovers — sprinkle this on anything you might be tempted to eat before carrying it back to the kitchen sink.

Serves 4
Preparation time 15 minutes, plus chilling
Cooking time 25 minutes

Nutritional values
Calories 135
Kilojoules 567
Protein 20 g
Carbohydrates 1 g
Fat 6 g

Tempeh balti

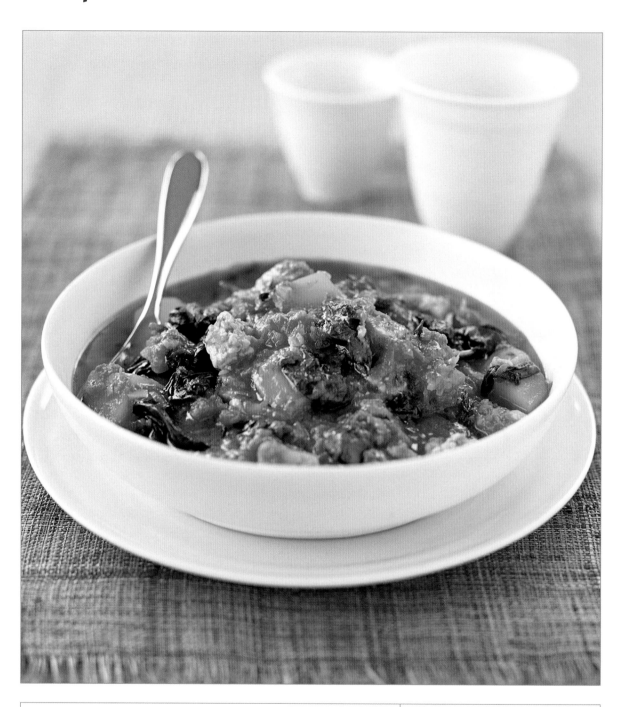

Serves 4
Preparation time 10 minutes
Cooking time 30 minutes

Nutritional values
Calories 376
Kilojoules 1579
Protein 20 g
Carbohydrates 40 g
Fat 14 g

8 oz tempeh, cut into $^1/_2$ inch cubes

3 garlic cloves, crushed

1 inch piece of fresh ginger root, grated

2 onions, roughly chopped

6 cardamom pods

2 teaspoons cumin

2 teaspoons coriander seeds

3 tablespoons groundnut or soy bean oil

2 cinnamon sticks

2 bay leaves

6 whole cloves

1 red chili, seeded and chopped

$^1/_2$ teaspoon turmeric

2 x 13 oz cans chopped tomatoes

2 teaspoons superfine sugar

1 lb potatoes, cut into cubes

8 oz spinach

1 Mix the tempeh in a bowl with the garlic and ginger. Blend the onions and 2 tablespoons water to a purée in a food processor.

2 Lightly crush the cardamom pods with the cumin and coriander with a mortar and pestle. Alternatively, put them in a plastic bag and crush to a fine powder with the back of a spoon.

3 Heat the oil in a large, nonstick pan and fry the crushed spices with the cinnamon, bay leaves, and cloves for 30 seconds. Tip the onion purée into the pan and add the chili and turmeric. Cook for 1 minute, then add the tomatoes, sugar, and potatoes and cover. Simmer gently for 20 minutes until the potatoes are tender and the sauce is thick. Add the tempeh and cook for a further 5 minutes.

4 Add the spinach to the pan, stirring it into the sauce until it starts to wilt. Cook for a further 2 minutes or until the spinach is soft and coated with the sauce. Serve immediately.

Don't serve yourself

If you are eating with the family, do not put food in serving dishes on the table — we tend to serve ourselves far more when we do this — not to mention the temptation to go for seconds. Serve things individually, not forgetting to reduce your plate size so that you don't over-indulge.

Diet-friendly food

This recipe contains many weight-loss friendly foods. Firstly, tempeh is made from soy paste which alters the way your body metabolizes fat, making weight loss easier. The dish also contains high levels of spicy herbs and flavorings. These have been proven to stimulate the production of endorphins and adrenaline in the body raising metabolic rate by as much as 25 percent after you've eaten them. A lot of the recipes in the diet are spicy for this purpose but there's nothing to stop you adding your own hot spices like chili, mustard, wasabi, or Tabasco to any meal you choose.

Liver with leeks and cannellini beans

4 pieces of calf's liver, about 4 oz each

4 tablespoons seasoned flour

4 teaspoons olive oil

4 large leeks, trimmed and sliced

4 lean Canadian bacon slices, chopped

1 lb canned cannellini beans, rinsed
   and drained

4 tablespoons sour cream

pepper

chopped parsley or thyme, to garnish

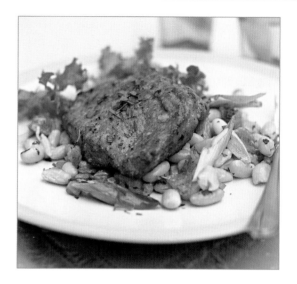

1 Toss the liver in the seasoned flour until evenly coated. Heat half the oil in a large, nonstick skillet, add the liver and fry for 2 minutes on each side or until cooked to your liking. Remove from the pan and keep warm.

2 Heat the remaining oil in the skillet, add the leeks and bacon and cook for 3–4 minutes. Stir in the cannellini beans and sour cream, season with pepper and heat through. Serve immediately, garnished with chopped parsley or thyme.

Serves 4
Preparation time 5 minutes
Cooking time 10 minutes

Nutritional values
Calories 389
Kilojoules 1630
Protein 39 g
Carbohydrates 39 g
Fat 11 g

Moussaka

12 oz new potatoes

1 teaspoon olive oil

1 large eggplant, chopped

12 oz lean ground lamb

1 onion, chopped

13 oz can chopped tomatoes

2 tablespoons tomato paste

1 teaspoon chopped oregano

4 oz feta cheese, crumbled

3 tablespoons low-fat plain yogurt

2 egg yolks, beaten

salt and pepper

1 Put the potatoes in a saucepan of boiling water and cook for 12–15 minutes until tender. Drain and slice.

2 Meanwhile, heat the oil in a large, nonstick skillet, add the eggplant and fry for 5 minutes. Add the ground lamb and onion and continue to fry for 5 minutes until the lamb is browned.

3 Add the potatoes, tomatoes, tomato paste and oregano, season to taste, bring to a boil and simmer for 15 minutes. Transfer the mixture to an ovenproof dish and keep warm.

4 Mix together the feta, yogurt, and egg yolks and pour over the meat mixture. Place under a preheated hot broiler for 3–4 minutes until golden and bubbling. Serve immediately.

What color is your kitchen?

Strange but true —the color of your kitchen could influence how much you eat. Yellow is particularly worrisome, as it stimulates appetite, but purple makes us headstrong and red can make us irritable and angry (triggering comfort binges). Good shades are green or pink, but the most appetite-suppressing color is blue. If you don't fancy a complete renovation, at least choose a blue tablecloth and/or plates — or put up a mirror so that you can see yourself eating. This cuts calorie intake by around 32 percent in trials.

Eat with your family

Need some encouragement to cook up one of the recipes here tonight? Research in the *American Journal of Clinical Nutrition* found that people eat less when they sit as a family and eat as a sense of occasion, rather than just eating for the sake of eating. Preparing something that looks amazing (like the Liver and Leeks dish featured here) could mean that you take your time over your meal and feel more satisfied.

Serves 4
Preparation time 10 minutes
Cooking time 35 minutes

Nutritional values
Calories 348
Kilojoules 1461
Protein 27 g
Carbohydrates 21 g
Fat 17 g

1
2
3
4
5

Evening snack

On the face of it, adding a sixth eating opportunity to the day, particularly in the hours before bed can seem extremely over-indulgent — after all, you will have been eating on and off all day. But when it comes to losing weight, this could be the most important meal you eat all day.

Your evening snack will give your metabolic rate a gentle nudge before you retire to sleep, and help combat the habit of nibbling empty calories that many of us indulge in during the evening before bed. By having a structured evening snack you won't feel the need to nibble all night to pass the time and you can fulfill your sugar craving in a measured dose. This naturally cuts down on your evening calories.

In trials at Wayne State University in the US, it was discovered that adding a snack of cereal and milk 90 minutes after an evening meal actually cut the energy intake of dieters by 400 calories (1680 kilojoules) a day, since they didn't feel the need to nibble as the night progressed. The other benefit of eating your snack 1–2 hours after your evening meal is that you will be feeling fairly full from your dinner. It actually takes 20 minutes to feel full after eating, but many of us eat dessert well before this. The result is that we don't realize how satisfied we actually are from our main meal, which causes us to eat more than we need.

It is once again important that you don't over-indulge with your evening snack — a small treat of around 100 calories is perfect and won't leave you bloated before bed which can be uncomfortable.

Choose from 40 snacks

The snacks here fall into two types: these two pages contain snacks to choose if you have trouble sleeping at night. They are full of sleep-inducing ingredients and easy to digest. Pages 112–113 contain snacks to choose if you'd prefer your evening snack to fulfil the role of dessert. Choose whichever you feel best fits your needs and mood, but if you haven't managed to meet your five portions of fruit and vegetables in any given day, do try to up the quota with your night-time choice.

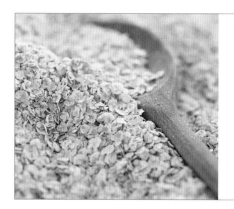

1 ¹/₂ cup **rolled oats** mixed as directed with ¹/₂ cup skim or soy milk. Add a spinkle of nutmeg before serving.

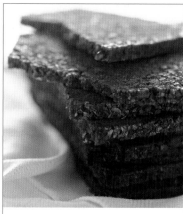

2 Half an **apple** spread with 1 teaspoon of peanut butter.

3 Half a **banana** and 4 Brazil nuts.

4 Two pieces of multigrain or **rye toast**.

5 One **cereal bar** (under 100 calories).

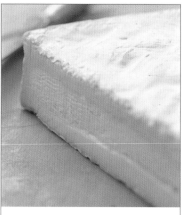

6 1 oz **brie cheese** on 2 water crackers.

WHY SLEEP IS SO IMPORTANT TO WEIGHT LOSS

A study in the *International Journal of Obesity* revealed that those who sleep nine hours a night are less likely to be overweight than those sleeping six hours a night. Fatigue seems to increase the amount of the fat-storage hormone insulin in the system, plus it reduces levels of the hormone leptin that tells you when you are full. It is easy to see how these two together can lead to weight gain. We are also more prone to sugar cravings when tired as the body tries to replenish the energy that it is lacking.

Trying to get eight hours' sleep a night is therefore important when you are dieting — and the foods you eat can play a part by delivering sleep-inducing chemicals or relaxing vitamins and minerals to your brain and body. Good choices include bananas (which have high levels of sedating magnesium); dairy products, which contain muscle-relaxing calcium; lettuce, which contains a sedative called lactucarium; foods such as turkey, avocado, or peanut butter that help the body to make a sleep-inducing substance called tryptophan; and pure carbohydrate foods like bread or jelly which cause rapid serotonin production that makes you sleepy.

7 Two tablespoons of **breakfast cereal** (non-sugary varieties like plain bran flakes are best) topped with a splash of skim or soy milk.

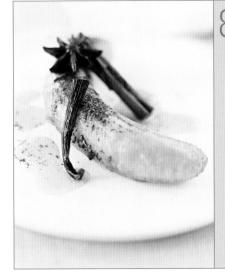

8 One serving of **Banana en Papillote** (see recipe on page 114). If this seems like too much effort to make in the evening, you can try slicing a banana and just sprinkling with a little cinnamon before eating.

THE NICEST WAY TO BURN CALORIES THIS EVENING

Do something that makes you laugh — according to research from Vanderbilt University in the US, laughing for 15 minutes each day burns 40 calories, which adds up to an additional weight loss of 4 lb over a year. While the obvious way to jolly things up in your evening is to watch something funny on the television, also try to think away from the box (so you're not tempted by all those fast-food ads). Think about visiting your local comedy club, calling a particularly witty friend, or even just lying in bed with a book that makes you laugh.

9 **Hot chocolate** made from 3/4 cup warmed skim or soy milk mixed with 1 envelope of low-calorie chocolate drink.

10 One small **brown or wholewheat roll** spread with a little yeast spread.

11 Two slices of deli **turkey**, each wrapped around a small slice of avocado.

12 4 oz low-fat **rice pudding**, add a little cinnamon on the top if you like it.

13 Half a **hot cross bun** spread with a scraping of low-fat spread.

14 One **chocolate-covered plain cookie** with 1/3 cup skim or soy milk.

15 125 g (4 oz) serving **crème caramel**.

16 One **peach** , sliced and served with 1/4 cup low -fat cottage cheese.

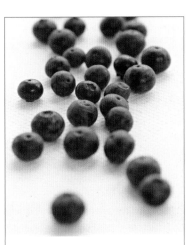

17 3 oz canned **tuna** in brine, served in 2 curled lettuce leaves.

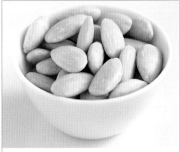

18 Five **almonds** mixed into a small carton of of low-fat yogurt or fromage frais.

19 One **Sesame Seed Oatcake** (see recipe on page 117) topped with 1 teaspoon of honey.

20 One tablespoon of **blueberries** mixed into 1 tablespoon low-fat plain yogurt served with a meringue nest.

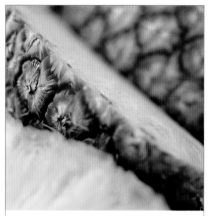

BEWARE FULL-MOON EATING
Research from Georgia State University in the US has found that people eat more on full-moon nights than normal. We don't know why, but the good news is that many astrologers believe the time of a waning moon that follows the full moon is one of the best times in the month to start a diet plan as the body enters elimination mode.

21 Two slices of fresh **pineapple**, broiled.

22 **Smoothie** of $^1/_2$ cup strawberries mixed with $^3/_4$ cup skim or soy milk and 1 teaspoon of cocoa powder.

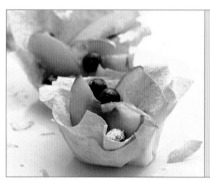

23 One **Mini Nectarine and Blueberry Tartlet** (see recipe on page 120). Accompany this with 2 teaspoons of low-fat yogurt or fromage frais.

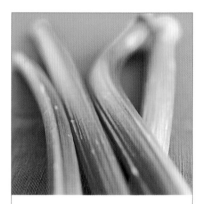

24 One individual carton of low-sugar **jello** or a 7 oz serving if you are making your own from gelatin dessert mix, topped with 1 tablespoon of reduced-fat light cream or a small squirt of aerosol cream.

25 1 oz scoop of **malted hot drink** powder, prepared as directed with $^1/_2$ cup skim milk and enough water to create your preferred thickness.

26 4 oz **rhubarb** stewed until soft, add $^1/_2$ teaspoon of sweetener and 2 tablespoons of low-fat yogurt.

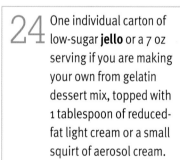

27 One small **chocolate ice cream bar** (about 1 oz).

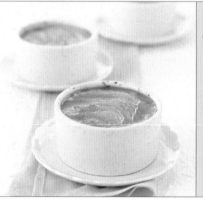

28 One **Mango and Passionfruit Brûlée** (see recipe on page 116). You could also try this recipe with 1 large peach or 5–6 apricots instead of mango.

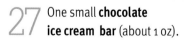

29 One carton of low-fat **chocolate mousse** (under 100 calories).

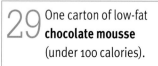

30 One individual carton (around 5 oz) low-fat **custard**.

31 Four medium-sized **marshmallow candies**.

QUICK QUESTION

I suffer from heartburn and find I can't eat late at night. Should I skip the snack?

Ideally not. Heartburn tends to occur if you eat large amounts or spicy foods late at night. As the portions here are small you may find it won't affect you, especially if you choose the blander evening meals. Other ways to reduce risk are sleeping on your left side and raising the upper half of your body by sleeping on extra pillows.

Ensuring your nightclothes are not too tight around the waist can also help reduce symptoms (too-tight waistbands push the contents of the stomach upward). If you still suffer, however, then skip the evening snack. The extra calories you could eat the next day when you're tired will far exceed the metabolic boost you get from eating this one final treat.

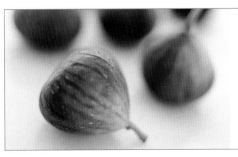

32 Two **fresh figs** served with 2 tablespoons ricotta or mascarpone cheese.

33 One **banana**, frozen then sliced and dipped in 1 teaspoon of honey.

34 3 oz serving of low-fat **vanilla ice cream**.

35 Two **rye crackers** spread with 2 teaspoons of low-sugar jelly.

36 **Brandy snap** filled with 1¹/₂ tablespoons low-fat yogurt and topped with 2 handfuls of raspberries.

37 One serving of **Fruit Kebabs with Strawberry Sauce** (see recipe on page 118).

38 One serving of **Mixed Fruit Sabayon** (see recipe on page 121).

39 Three wafer thin **after-dinner mints**.

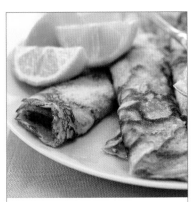

40 One **lemon crêpe** (around 1 ¹/₂ oz) topped with 1 teaspoon low-fat vanilla ice cream.

SO YOU HAD A BAD DAY

Spending five minutes before bed thinking about how well your diet went today can help ensure success. But what if things didn't go so well? Don't give up; this five-point plan will help you get back on the wagon tomorrow.

1 Get a pen and paper and choose all your meals and snacks for tomorrow; make them things you know you can eat. There's no point wanting pancakes for breakfast if you only have cereal in the cupboard.

2 Think about what went wrong today and why. When you've worked out why, write down three ways you could avoid it happening again.

3 Set your alarm for 20 minutes earlier than normal tomorrow morning for a walk before breakfast. This will help reinforce your commitment to the diet plan and help you wear off some of the calories you consumed today.

4 Go to bed and forget completely about today. Other than your walk tomorrow morning, you're not going to try and make up for it in any way.

5 After your walk eat the breakfast you planned and really focus on sticking to your plan for the rest of the day.

Evening snack recipes

If you find that you eat in the evening to pass the time, use that time to create some of these recipes — just watch that you don't consume extra calories while preparing the dish. Finally, remember the first three recipes contain ingredients prized for their sleep-inducing abilities, while the second three are more suitable for those with a seriously sweet tooth.

Banana en papillote

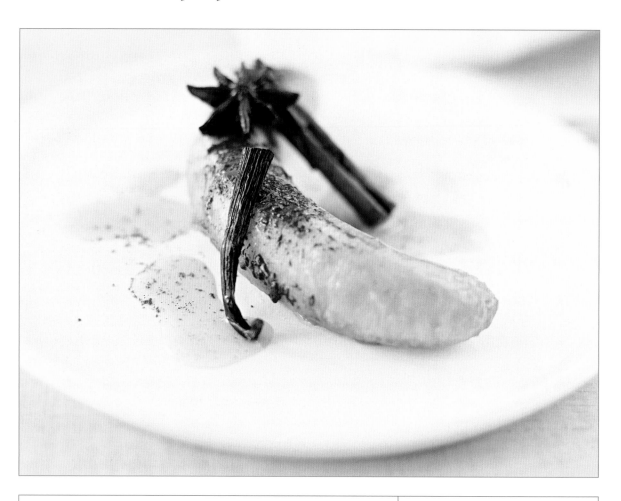

Serves 4
Preparation time 2 minutes
Cooking time 3 minutes

Nutritional values
Calories 126
Kilojoules 529
Protein 2 g
Carbohydrates 30 g
Fat 0 g

oil, for cooking

4 small, firm bananas

1 cinnamon stick, cut into 4

4 star anise

1 vanilla bean, cut into 4

2 tablespoons grated carob

$1/3$ cup pineapple juice

1 Lightly grease 4 pieces of kitchen foil or waxed paper, each large enough to wrap around a banana. Place a banana in the center and add a piece of cinnamon, 1 star anise, and a piece of vanilla bean.

2 Sprinkle with grated carob and pineapple juice and fold over the foil to make an airtight pocket.

3 Place the sealed bananas on a baking sheet and cook in a preheated oven, 450°F, for 3–4 minutes. Serve immediately.

Top banana

Not only are bananas weight-loss-friendly fruits that help you sleep, they are also one of the best dietary sources of potassium which helps the body regulate fluid intake. Women are prone to fluid retention, which adds extra pounds on the scales and inches to the waistline. Increasing the amount of potassium foods like bananas and other good sources like sweet potatoes, tomatoes, and peaches in your diet, and decreasing the amount of salt you consume, will help flush out this extra fluid and speed up your weight-loss efforts.

Do you have night-eating syndrome (NES)?

This rare condition was first identified in the 1950s and affects 1.5 percent of the population. The problem is characterized by the need to eat excessively between the hours of 8 p.m. and 6.a.m. Some people even find they have to get up in the middle of the night so they can eat. While it's believed the problem is linked to abnormal hormone levels (particularly low levels of melatonin that makes us sleep and leptin that makes us hungry), new research has found the problem is strongly related to stress. If you have this problem, you could be affected by NES and will benefit from looking at ways to get your stress levels under control. In trials at the Medical University of South Carolina, NES sufferers who started 20 minutes of meditation a day experienced a reduction in symptoms in as little as a week.

Mango and passionfruit brûlée

1 small mango, peeled and thinly sliced

2 passionfruit, flesh scooped out

1¹/₄ cup low-fat plain yogurt

³/₄ cup sour cream

1 tablespoon confectioners' sugar

few drops of vanilla extract

2 tablespoons raw sugar

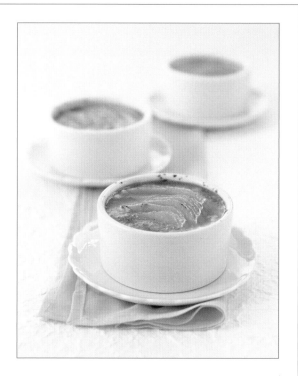

1 Divide the mango slices equally among 4 ramekins.

2 Stir together the passionfruit flesh, yogurt, sour cream, and confectioners' sugar and spoon over the mango. Tap the ramekins to give a flat surface.

3 Sprinkle over the raw sugar and cook under a preheated hot broiler for 1–2 minutes until the sugar is melted. Chill for 30 minutes before serving.

Serves 4
Preparation time 10 minutes, plus chilling
Cooking time 2 minutes

Nutritional values
Calories 131
Kilojoules 550
Protein 5 g
Carbohydrates 19 g
Fat 5 g

Sesame seed oatcakes

1 cup oatmeal

1 tablespoon sesame seeds

pinch of salt

pinch of baking soda

1 tablespoon olive oil

2–3 tablespoons hot water

1 Mix together all the ingredients in a bowl to form a firm dough, adding a little water if necessary. The mixture will be very crumbly so just keep pressing it back together.

2 Roll out the mixture on a lightly floured surface as thinly as you can. Cut 12 triangles or 3 inch rounds and place them on cookie sheets.

3 Bake in a preheated oven, 350°F, for about 10 minutes until golden and firm. Cool on a wire rack. The oatcakes can be stored in an airtight container for up to 3 days.

Five tactics to fight refrigerator-raiding

If you find yourself aimlessly wandering to the refrigerator even after your evening snack, try these five tactics to stop putting those mindless calories in your mouth:

1 Write motivational messages like "you can do this" on bright pieces of paper and stick them at eye level on the refrigerator. The color will break through your consciousness and the messages will help your motivation.

2 Turn up the lights. Doctors at California State University have found that we eat more in darker rooms as our inhibitions are dimmed.

3 Some joke stores sell dancing plants or oinking pigs that respond to light. Buy one and place it in the refrigerator; as the door opens it will attract your attention.

4 Stick tape across the entrance to the kitchen to stop you entering.

5 Store all "snack" foods in containers with tight lids; you'll soon realize what you're doing as you find yourself struggling to get the lids off.

Makes 12
Preparation time 10 minutes
Cooking time 10 minutes

Nutritional values
Calories 79
Kilojoules 330
Protein 2 g
Carbohydrates 11 g
Fat 3 g

Fruit kebabs with strawberry sauce

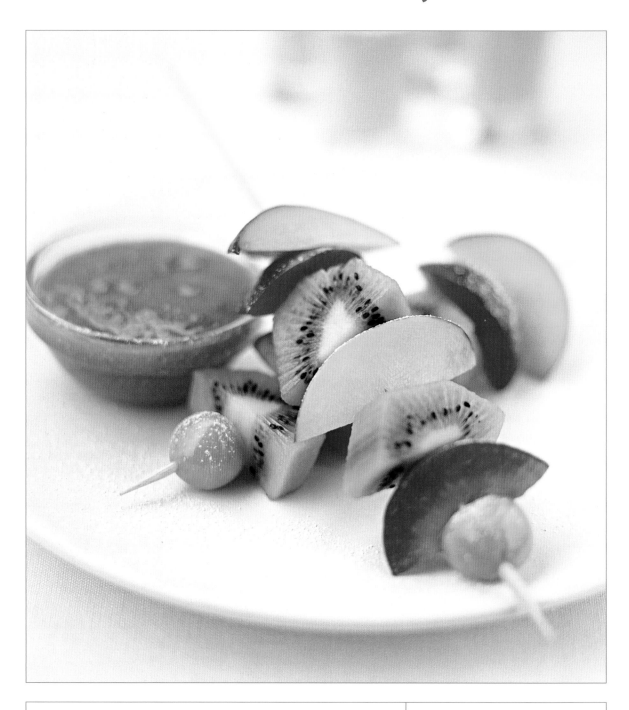

Serves 4
Preparation time 5 minutes
Cooking time 2–3 minutes

Nutritional values
Calories 109
Kilojoules 457
Protein 3 g
Carbohydrates 26 g
Fat 0 g

1 lb firm mixed fruit (such as kiwifruit, nectarines, and melon)

2^1/$_2$ cups strawberries

^{2}/$_3$ cup orange juice

1 Cut the fruit into large cubes. Thread the pieces onto kebab sticks and broil for 2–3 minutes under a preheated hot broiler, turning occasionally.

2 Meanwhile, make the sauce. Blend the strawberries with the orange juice in a food processor until smooth. Dip the kebabs in the sauce and serve immediately.

Are you a happy eater?

Studies reveal that some mood states may make people more prone to night-time nibbling — women tend to eat when they are bored, depressed, or tired, while men tend to binge when they have had a good day and are happy or feel they deserve a reward. If you know your day may make you more prone to bingeing make sure that you have your non-food rewards or anti-refrigerator raiding tactics ready.

The early bird loses the weight

Night owls are more likely to overeat than those who go to bed early, says research from the University of California. The longer you are awake, the more nibbling opportunities you have. Adjusting your sleep schedule can therefore help you cut calories. If you find it hard to drop off early, here are some tips that can help:
• Avoid caffeine-containing drinks after lunch; caffeine can take over ten hours to leave the system.
• Make sure your bedroom is dark; light pollution from street lights or blinking clock alarms can suppress the production of the sleep hormone melatonin in some people.
• Have a hot bath before bed. The body is stimulated to sleep by a fall in temperature and the rapid cooling that occurs after a hot bath mimics this in the body.
• Add some jasmine or lavender oils to the bath. Both of these have been shown to make it easier for people to fall asleep and stay asleep for longer once they do.

Nectarine and blueberry tartlets

oil, for brushing

4 sheets of phyllo pastry (thawed if frozen), each 12 x 7 inches

2 tablespoons low-sugar red berry jelly

juice of $^1/_2$ orange

4 ripe nectarines, halved, pitted, and sliced

1 cup blueberries

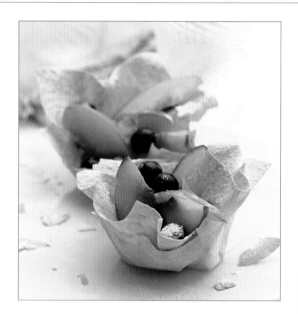

1 Lightly oil the sheets of phyllo pastry and cut each into 6 pieces, each 4 x $3^1/_2$ inches. Arrange a piece in each of the sections of a deep, lightly oiled, 12-hole muffin pan. Add a second piece at a slight angle to the first to give a pretty, jagged edge to each pastry shell.

2 Bake the tartlets in a preheated oven, 350°F, for 6–8 minutes until golden.

3 Meanwhile, warm the jelly and orange juice in a large saucepan, add the nectarines and blueberries and warm through.

4 Carefully lift the tartlet shells out of the muffin pan and transfer them to a serving dish. Fill with the warm fruits and serve.

Makes 12
Preparation time 15 minutes
Cooking time 6–8 minutes

Nutritional values
Calories 75
Kilojoules 310
Protein 1 g
Carbohydrates 9 g
Fat 4 g

Mixed fruit sabayon

4 fresh apricots, halved, pitted, and sliced

1$\frac{1}{3}$ cups strawberries, halved or quartered (depending on size)

1 cup seedless red grapes, halved if large

2 kiwifruit, each peeled and cut into 8 long, thin slices

2 egg yolks

2 tablespoons superfine sugar

5 tablespoons sparkling white grape and elderflower juice

1 Mix the fruit together and divide among 4 shallow, ovenproof dishes.

2 Half-fill a saucepan with water, bring to a boil and put a large bowl over the top, checking that the base of the bowl does not touch the water. Add the egg yolks, sugar, and juice to the bowl and beat, using a whisk or electric beater, for 4–5 minutes until the mixture is thick and frothy and leaves a peak when the beater is lifted.

3 Pour the frothy custard over the fruits and place under a hot preheated broiler for 1–2 minutes until just browned. Serve immediately.

Light and flaky

Phyllo pastry is one of the healthy exchanges dieters can make to ensure they enjoy foods like fruit tarts without ruining their diets. At 300 calories (1260 kj) per 3 $\frac{1}{2}$ oz compared with puff pastry at 400 calories (1680 kj) for the same amount, these phyllo tarts won't put a dent in your daily calorie budget. Other healthy swaps include choosing soft cheese over hard, bread crumbs instead of batter, picking white meat or fish dishes over those based on red meat and switching full-fat versions of foods like milk, spreads, potato chips, cookies in your diet for their reduced-fat versions.

Serves 4
Preparation time 15 minutes
Cooking time 5–7 minutes

Nutritional values
Calories 130
Kilojoules 546
Protein 3 g
Carbohydrates 43 g
Fat 3 g

Maintaining your weight

So you know exactly how to lose the weight with this little-and-often diet but what happens when the diet is over? Just how do you keep those pounds from creeping back on. That is where the tips and tricks you've learned while following the plan can help.

It is an annoying quirk of biology that as you lose weight, you'll actually burn fewer calories a day than you did at your old weight. This is partly down to the body's natural conservation tactics, which slows the metabolic rate a little to try and regain the fat it has lost; but also because the less you weigh, the less effort it takes to move around and so the less calories you burn doing it. Circumventing these changes is the key to keeping off

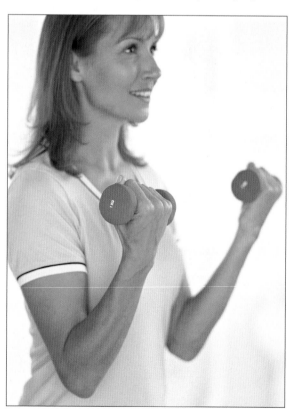

the weight you've lost and here are a number of ways you can do this:

1 Eat at least three small meals and two snacks a day. This will naturally keep your metabolism running at the highest rate possible throughout the day and also prevent hunger pangs and sugar cravings that can lead to excessive snacking.

2 Try to increase the amount of muscle you possess. Muscles burn more calories than fat, even at rest, so the more of it you have the faster your metabolism runs. The best way to build muscle is strength-training; try to do three 30-minute sessions a week, either at the gym or by buying a set of hand weights and a good exercise video.

3 Eat the right number of calories for your body. See the box opposite to work this out.

4 Keep portion sizes small; allowing larger servings of food to creep onto your plate is the most common reason people regain their weight. If you find that you're feeling bloated after eating, or start to lose interest in a dish halfway through it's likely that you are serving yourself too much.

5 Choose low GI foods wherever possible. As well as lowering insulin levels, picking wholegrains over carbohydrates actually revs up the metabolic rate enough to prevent a weight gain of almost 8 lb a year.

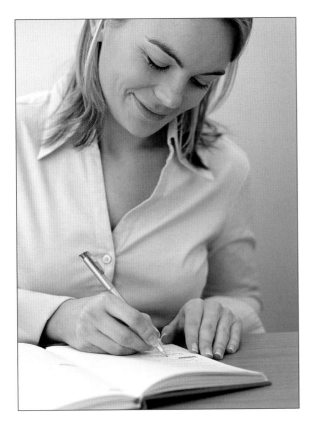

Also, lower your GI intake by trying to eat a little protein at most meals and snacks, and making the fruit or vegetable part of your meal the largest part instead of carbohydrates.

6 Keep a food diary for a few days a month to try to spot any extra calories creeping in. Remember, prime points for invisible calories are when cooking, when clearing up leftovers, and while standing over the refrigerator deciding exactly what to have for dinner that evening.

7 Don't fixate over every fluctuation. Regular eating patterns create a far healthier metabolic profile than days where you eat erratically, so starving just because the scales say you're $2^1/_4$ lb heavier today, could actually trigger more problems than it solves. If the scales go up a bit don't worry about it, unless it does it consistently for four days or more (and, if you are female those four days are not the ones just prior to your period). Only adjust your eating when weight gain looks set to stay put — then just go back on the plan for a week or two to sort things out and remind yourself just how good healthy eating can taste.

Calculate how many calories you need each day

This is determined by how much you weigh in relation to your height and the amount of activity you do each day:

1 Multiply your weight in pounds by ten (to work out calories) or your weight in kilograms by 92.4 (to calculate kilojoules).

2 Now multiply this by the number in front of the description below that sounds most like your activity level:

- Multiply by 1.3 if you have a sedentary job and do no or only a little gentle exercise.

- Multiply by 1.4 if you have a moderately active job (shopworker or home maker) or exercise moderately (walking or social swimming) for at least 30 minutes a day.

- Multiply by 1.5 if you have a fairly active job (postperson, police officer) or exercise hard for more than 30 minutes a day.

- Multiply by 1.7 if you have a very active job (builder or personal trainer), or work out intensely for more than an hour a day.

Questions and answers

Still confused about how this little-and-often eating plan can fit into your life? Here are some answers to some of the questions that could come up as you give the plan a try.

I don't like one of the ingredients in a meal you've suggested. Can I change things?
Yes; this isn't a diet that relies on strange food combinations to work. However, you do need to swap like for like (a protein like fish can be swapped for another protein like chicken, seafood, tofu, or lean steak, while a carbohydrate like rice can be swapped for pasta), and keep portion sizes the same.

I work shifts so how do I make everything fit around them?
Try to eat the meal you should be eating naturally at this point in your sleep/wake cycle; for example, when you wake up, eat breakfast even if it's 3 p.m. One change you should make is to add a small portion of protein (a couple of slices of turkey, a few almonds, or a few tablespoons of cottage cheese) to your afternoon snack. When you are tired your insulin response is incredibly sensitive to sugar, and some of the snacks here may cause too sudden a rise and the subsequent crash this triggers. Adding protein will prevent this.

I can't eat all that food in one day. I hardly eat anything at the moment.
You may be eating small meals, but they are probably high in fat which taxes your digestion, leaving you bloated. When you switch to the lower-fat, easier-to-digest meals here you may find your appetite increases. But to start with, choose meals that are easy to split in half, prepare it as directed but stop when you feel full and set the dish aside. If you get hungry again an hour later, finish it off. If not, just eat your next snack as planned. Your body will soon start to tell you what it needs.

My family eats at 6 p.m. — can I skip my afternoon snack?
No; remember, it is leaving too long between meals that causes the big problem not squishing them up. If you want to pull your afternoon snack forward to 3.30 then eat at 6 p.m. or have your evening snack at 8 p.m. so you can be in bed by 9 p.m. that's fine. Just remember to eat your breakfast as close to waking as you can.

I can't find anything I like in the morning snacks. Can I have two of the afternoon ones each day?
In terms of calories, it won't make any difference. But remember, the body functions best on the particular mixes of proteins and carbohydrates suggested for each time of day on the plan, so to truly get the most benefits it is best to try and find something you like from each section.

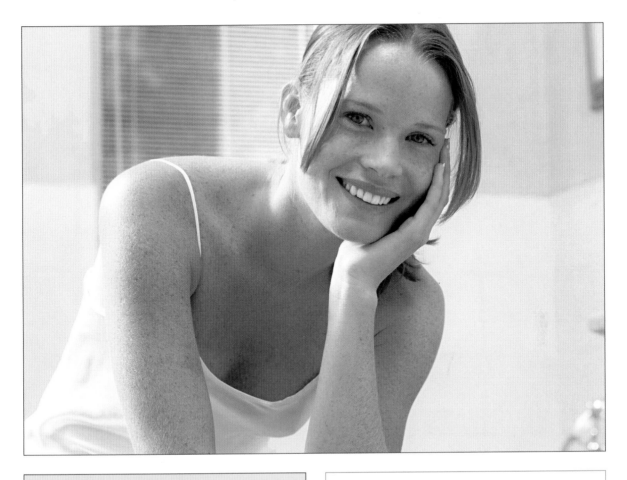

I'm not losing weight. What's wrong?

Assuming that you are not under 119 lb (in which case turn to pages 14–15), the most common reason is that invisible calories are creeping into your diet. Keep a food diary of every mouthful you eat to pinpoint danger times and watch those optional treats like the odd glass of wine or the extra snack. If you choose all of these you will consume more calories than you need and weight loss won't occur.

But I promise I have stuck to the guidelines and it's still not coming off?

In this case, particularly if you're suffering other symptoms such as fatigue, menstrual irregularities, or changes in hair growth (sudden loss or excess), then a medical condition like under-active thyroid or polycystic ovaries could be causing you problems. Ask your doctor for a check-up.

And what if I'm vegetarian — can I adapt the meat-based meals?

Yes, by adding a vegetable or meat substitute — for example, large mushrooms and thick lima beans make a great substitute for the beef in the Beef Ragout recipe on page 100, while switching the salami topping on the French Bread Pizzas on page 69 for artichoke hearts is a delicious alternative. Remember though, vegetables and even most meat substitutes contain less calories per ounce than meat does, so don't skimp on portions or you could end up cutting out too many calories. Ideally, add twice the weight if you're using solely vegetables or an extra third if you're using a higher protein alternative like beans or tofu or meat substitute.

Index

Acknowledgments

Executive Editor Nicky Hill
Editor Emma Pattison
Executive Art Editor Karen Sawyer
Designer Janis Utton
Jacket Designer Claire Legemah
Props stylist Liz Hippisley
Photographer Gareth Sambidge
Picture Librarian Sophie Delpech
Production Controller Nosheen Shan

Special photography: © Octopus Publishing Group Limited/Gareth Sambidge.

Other photography: DigitalVision 17. ImageSource 125. **Octopus Publishing Group Limited**/Frank Adam 42 top right, 44 top, 57 bottom, 78 top, 90 top, 111 bottom left; /Stephen Conroy 22, 26 top, 57 center left, 59 center left, 79 top, 112 center right; /Gus Filgate 113 bottom; /Jeremy Hopley 23 center right; /Sandra Lane 60 top, 60 center right, 94 bottom left, 95 bottom; /William Lingwood 23, 24 bottom left, 26 bottom left, 28, 34, 43, 45 center right, 46, 60 bottom left, 61 top, 70, 72, 78 bottom, 79 bottom, 84, 91 top, 93 top, 96, 100, 112 center left,

120; /Neil Mersh 27 center right; /Sean Myers 45 bottom left; /Lis Parsons 24 top, 24 bottom right, 26 bottom right, 27 center left, 38, 42 top left, 44 center left, 44 bottom, 50, 52, 57 top, 59 top, 61 center left, 62, 66, 76 top left, 76 bottom, 93 bottom, 95 top, 104, 112 bottom, 116; /Mike Prior 122; /Peter Pugh-Cook 13, 15; /William Reavell 45 top left, 56, 58 bottom left, 59 bottom right, 76 top right, 92 bottom, 110 top left, 110 top right; /Russell Sadur 8, 11; /Karen Thomas 25 bottom; /Unit Photographic 19; /Ian Wallace 23 center left, 42 bottom left, 43 bottom, 44 center right, 58 center, 91 bottom, 94 center right, 110 bottom, 111 bottom right. **PhotoDisc** 14.